Antenna

Related titles

FUNDAMENTALS OF OBSTETRICS AND GYNAECOLOGY
Fifth edition
Volume 1   Obstetrics
Volume 2   Gynaecology
Derek Llewellyn-Jones

ANATOMY AND PHYSIOLOGY OF OBSTETRICS
Sixth edition
Mary Anderson

MIDWIFERY QUESTIONS ANSWERED
Valerie Smith and the Tutors of Queen Charlotte's Hospital, London

AN A–Z OF GYNAECOLOGY
Mary Anderson

PREPARING FOR PREGNANCY
Philip J. Robarts

EVERYWOMAN: A GYNAECOLOGICAL GUIDE FOR LIFE
Fifth edition
Derek Llewellyn-Jones

PREGNANCY AFTER THIRTY
Mary Anderson

BREAST FEEDING: HOW TO SUCCEED
Derek Llewellyn-Jones

A CHILD IS BORN
Lennart Nilsson

Antenatal Teaching

A Guide to Theory and Practice

Patricia Wilson

SRN SCM

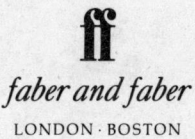

faber and faber

LONDON · BOSTON

First published in 1990
by Faber and Faber Limited
3 Queen Square London WC1N 3AU

Photoset by Parker Typesetting Service Leicester
Printed in Great Britain by
Richard Clay Ltd Bungay Suffolk

All rights reserved

© Patricia Wilson, 1990

This book is sold subject to the condition that it shall not, by way of trade or otherwise, be lent, resold, hired out or otherwise circulated without the publisher's prior consent in any form of binding or cover other than that in which it is published and without a similar condition including this condition being imposed on the subsequent purchaser

A CIP record for this book is available from the British Library.

ISBN 0 571 14113 7

To Eric, who first opened my eyes to the world of learning

Contents

Acknowledgements ix
Foreword xi
Introduction xiii

1 **Antenatal Education Goals** 1
   Aims; Objectives; Assessment; Evaluation.
2 **Theories of Learning** 13
   Motivation; How we learn; Factors that affect learning.
3 **Planning** 25
   Subject knowledge; Client need; Teaching methods; Group work; Teaching aids; Working with other people; Lesson plans; Checklist for planning.
4 **Partners** 55
   Partners' needs, their role in support during pregnancy, birth and after.
5 **Pregnancy** 71
   Fetal development; Nutrition; Tobacco, alcohol and drugs; Exercise and physical comfort; Emotions and sex in pregnancy; Antenatal care; Layette and baby equipment; Safety in the home; Car safety.
6 **Relaxation and Breathing for Labour** 93
   Choice of relaxation method; The Mitchell Method of Relaxation; Mental relaxation; Breathing in relaxation; Reasons for teaching breathing for labour; Choice of method of breathing for labour; Breathing for the first stage of labour; Breathing for the second stage of labour.

7 **Labour and Birth** 112
Signs of labour and admission to hospital;
Physiology of labour; Coping strategies; Pain relief;
Labour ward procedures and policies; Medical
intervention.

8 **Baby Care and Feeding** 140
Choice of feeding method; Advantages and
disadvantages of feeding methods; Theory and
practice of breastfeeding; Theory and practice of
bottlefeeding; Other practical feeding
considerations; Care of the baby by the mother;
Care of the baby by the midwife; Care of the baby
by the paediatrician.

9 **Life After Birth** 169
Physical needs and care in the puerperium;
Emotional and sexual needs in the puerperium;
Taking baby home; Role of the health visitor;
Postnatal examination.

Appendix 1   Resources 183
Appendix 2   What next? Suggestions for further study 192
Index 201

Acknowledgements

My thanks to Kathy Lacy, Health Education Officer, for being a wise and sympathetic sounding board for my ideas; to Val Box and the tutors on the Health Education Certificate course, a project for which was the basis of this book; to Margie Polden, Obstetric Physiotherapist, for all I have learned from her and for her comradeship over the years; to Margaret Adams, whose advice, encouragement and enthusiasm kept me going; to Roger Osborne of Faber and Faber for his patient guidance of a novice author; and to Barbara Jones, my manager at Hammersmith Hospital, for her support. Thanks to my colleagues who took the time and trouble to offer constructive criticism of the manuscript. It is impossible to thank by name all the tutors, colleagues and clients from whom I have learned and continue to learn. Finally, thanks to my family for their patience; they have suffered in the process of getting this book to press.

The Mitchell Method of Relaxation, extracted from *Simple Relaxation* by Laura Mitchell, is published by permission of the author and John Murray (Publishers) Ltd.

The information on the City and Guilds of London Course 7307, Further and Adult Education Teachers' Certificate, is taken from the pamphlet issued by the Institute and is published with their permission.

The cartoons are by Ros Asquith from her book *Baby* and are reproduced by kind permission of Ros Asquith and Macdonald-Optima publishers.

Foreword

Antenatal teaching in modern society, which has high expectations of the experience of childbirth and parenthood, is often a daunting task. Many midwives and other professionals are ill-prepared for this role. Priority is sometimes given to imparting information about material facilities and support available for the parents. This is useful but may be at the expense of helping with the social and the psychological adjustment needed in the transition into parenthood.

Parents are the most diverse group of people to be educated, since they may be from any social position, any educational and any cultural background that is in the locality. In order to attempt to meet their many varied needs, a move away from the didactic approach is necessary. Many educators, however, lack the expertise and skills needed to facilitate confidently client-centred groups. This very comprehensive book provides resources for anyone who wishes to change or improve and enrich their teaching skills. Throughout this book the experience and philosophy of the author is evident. She clearly demonstrates her own commitment to thinking of the group's priorities rather than those of the educator, and to meet, wherever possible, the needs of the individual member.

This book also contains a wealth of information which will be of use to all who are in contact with, or caring for, clients going through the process of becoming parents.

Margaret Adams
MSc SRN SCM DN MTD

Introduction

This book is designed to give midwives, health visitors and others an insight into antenatal education. It is especially aimed at those who are expected to teach antenatal classes before undertaking formal training in this field. It is not intended to replace parentcraft teaching or health education courses, but rather to provide a lifeline to those teachers who are thrown in at the deep end. It will not necessarily provide answers, but rather food for thought, some alternative methods to consider and possible resources to tap.

There is a large amount of literature available which is useful for those who are, or wish to become, antenatal teachers. There are books giving information about the subjects taught in antenatal classes and there are books on education theory and practice. I have attempted to draw together the essentials: some theories on learning and teaching and some methods that can be employed, relating these to the field of antenatal education; providing material that can be easily assimilated and giving a sound educational basis on which teachers may build their practice.

My own experience as a midwife and antenatal teacher is that many midwives are ill-prepared to teach antenatal classes when they begin the job. Most training takes place 'in post'. Limited availability of finance often delays the training of teachers and some antenatal teachers continue to teach without training. I believe that a book which provides basic guidance in an easily digestible form can play a useful role. It is only an introduction and further training will be needed.

A small survey of twenty-eight midwives was carried out in

Introduction

February/March 1987. A questionnaire was sent to midwives currently engaged in antenatal education. The results supported my hypothesis that the majority of midwives who began antenatal teaching did so before undertaking any specific training for the job.

82 per cent commenced teaching without attending a teaching course.
46 per cent commenced teaching without any tuition in the theories of learning or practical planning of antenatal classes.
29 per cent had never received any tuition, either during midwifery training, or before or since commencing teaching.
32 per cent had attended a course only after commencing teaching.

These findings support a paper by Trisha Black[1] which reported the results of courses held in Blackburn in 1982 and Blackburn and South East Wales in 1983, the course participants being midwives and health visitors. Of the midwives questioned, 33 per cent of those who had undergone twelve-month training and 23 per cent of those who had undergone eighteen-month training felt unprepared to undertake antenatal teaching. Health visitors had more emphasis on education during training but were not always midwives. Those that were soon felt out of date regarding hospital practices. Course participants were equally divided between midwives and health visitors. Twenty-five per cent had no previous teaching experience. Twenty-five per cent had some previous training: City and Guilds of London Course 7307, Further and Adult Education Teachers' Certificate, Health Education Certificate or other training.

This book aims to bridge the gap that often occurs between commencing teaching and formal training. It does not aim to be prescriptive. The intention is not to set down what or how you should teach your clients; rather you are invited to consider what you are trying to do, some alternative ways of

Introduction

achieving your goals and how you evaluate the results. You are also invited to consider what educational psychologists, teachers, researchers and others have learned and how that can have a bearing on your own work.

There is no foolproof plan, no programme which will guarantee success. This book does not set down a course of antenatal classes. You will need to discover what is right for you and for your clients, in the particular situation in which you are teaching. Many hospitals or districts provide guidelines for their antenatal teachers and this book seeks to supplement such guidelines. Teachers, courses and clients will vary.

Since most mothers are delivered in hospital, the book is written with this in mind. However, much of the content is valid for midwives preparing mothers to deliver at home.

The first three chapters form the basis for planning antenatal teaching. First, you are asked to consider your goals. The process of constructing aims and objectives will help you to clarify precisely what you are trying to do. If antenatal education is viewed in the broader context of health education, teaching can be planned to take in the wider issues of an individual's right and responsibility to maintain her own and her family's health. It follows that when you have decided what you wish to do, you need to be able to assess and evaluate your work. Ways of measuring your achievement of your aims and objectives are suggested, as are methods of evaluating the success of your teaching strategies and the usefulness of the learning to the clients.

Second, some theories of learning are considered. Teachers can be more effective if they understand why and how people learn and what may hinder the learning process. It is also important to consider the relationships that are formed between teacher and learner and the perceptions they have of one another.

Third, the planning of content and strategies is discussed. The subjects traditionally taught in antenatal classes are likely to be of interest to clients, and note should be taken of clients'

Introduction

views. Different teaching methods are listed and their use in antenatal classes is considered. You are asked to take account of practical details in the planning of sessions; lesson plans, teaching notes, venue, seating arrangements, teaching aids and working in conjunction with other teachers, both lay and professional.

Chapter 4 discusses the partner's role, both from the viewpoint of how he can help the mother and how he can be helped to cope with the change to fatherhood. This area is often neglected in antenatal teaching.

Chapters 5–9 cover the commonly taught subjects, and information can be extracted from one or several sections to help you plan your sessions. The division of subjects is to some extent arbitrary, as it is recognized that teachers will plan their courses in different ways.

In each chapter you are asked first to decide on your aims and objectives. Then you are asked to think about what material you will cover. Some suggestions are given, together with source references. A list of possible teaching aids is given. As encouraging client participation is often difficult for new teachers, some questions suitable for stimulating discussion are included. The need to assess and evaluate the session is emphasized.

The final section of the book covers resources, possible sources of information and teaching aids. Details are given of courses of study which will enable teachers to develop their skills.

The format of the material presented in the book is based on the premise that to be effective, learning needs to be active. I have therefore posed many questions, and rather than providing definitive answers have suggested some alternatives that will hopefully act as stimuli for readers to think for themselves. I have also attempted to stimulate thought by relating helpful and unhelpful teaching strategies to your own experiences. Readers are encouraged to use the suggestions made in the book, not merely accepting the ideas

Introduction

but critically evaluating all they do. The book is designed to encourage learning by experience and to stimulate further study and learning.

My experience in helping midwives develop their teaching skills has been that their knowledge of what they are teaching is good, and that they try to impart information in a way that their clients will understand. However, they often need assistance to look at their subject matter from the clients' point of view rather than from their own professional viewpoint, and insufficient thought is sometimes given to what exactly they are trying to do in antenatal education.

I hope that, using this book, midwives and others will come to a greater understanding of their goals and the factors which help or hinder learning. Experience gained from using different teaching methods and aids will enable them to judge what suits their own groups. Some readers may find their own work has already prepared them to cope with some of the aspects dicussed. I have tried to offer suggestions where standard midwifery training and experience may not provide relevant material. I hope this book will be used both as a starting point for beginners and as a reference for antenatal teachers to review their work.

Patricia Wilson, 1989

References

1 Black, T. (1986), *Antenatal Education: Teaching the Teachers*, Report of Seminar paper presented at the Health Education Council, London.

1
Antenatal Education Goals

As antenatal educators, you have a unique opportunity to influence not only how a mother copes with pregnancy and childbirth but also her future health and that of her family. Before deciding what you will teach you need to decide what you are trying to achieve, that is, you need to develop your aims and objectives. If you think of aims as the broad, overall view of what you hope your clients will achieve, and objectives as the specific, precise learning that you expect them to demonstrate, this will give you a working definition to help you plan your work.

You will need to make a judgement of whether your goals have been reached. Assessment and evaluation of your teaching will help you to decide this and also to plan more effectively in the future. Assessment is here taken to be judgement of what, and how much, the client has learned and how she has put her learning into practice. Evaluation is a judgement by the teacher of her own techniques and the effectiveness of the planning, content and strategies of her teaching.

1 Aims

The aims of antenatal education have changed. In the nineteenth century an effort was made to reduce high infant mortality by instructing mothers in good hygiene practices. Later, helping women to cope with the pain of childbirth was felt to be important. More recently the emphasis has been on emotional factors and teaching the necessary skills to cope with life changes.[1]

We can take the broader perspective and see antenatal education as part of health education. It is important to look at the ideologies and theories on which different models of health education are based.

One view of such models is as follows:

(a) Behavioural change – in which improvements in health are sought by facilitating a change in behaviour. For example, educating people to give up smoking.
(b) Self-empowerment – in which individuals are enabled to develop the ability to understand and control the determinants of health within possible economic or other constraints. For example, enabling women to maximize their chances of a normal and satisfying birth, taking into account both physical and emotional factors.
(c) Collective action – which seeks to improve health by bringing individuals together to strive for changes in environmental, social and economic factors. For example, working with the Association for Improvement in the Maternity Services (AIMS).[2]

Health education theories and practices are still developing and it is important for antenatal educators to be part of this field.

In the light of health education models, consider whether the aims for antenatal education should be emphasized in any of the following ways:

Enabling clients, through knowledge, to make health decisions for themselves.
Helping clients to become more aware of the influence they can have on the factors that contribute to a fulfilled life.
Assisting clients to gain or remain in control of their lives.
Persuading clients to make changes in their lifestyles that will improve their health.

Antenatal Education Goals

Do you believe health educators have the right to try to change people's behaviour? Do teachers know best what is good for clients? Medical knowledge is not complete, professionals do not always agree among themselves and fashions are always changing in the management of labour and care of babies. As antenatal educators we must equip ourselves with the most complete knowledge available, give our clients the best advice we believe in, but never lose sight of the individual's right and responsibility to maintain control of his or her own life.

To be useful, aims should be stated in terms of learner behaviour, not the activities or goals of the teacher. For example, the aim 'to teach parenting skills' says nothing about learner attainment. But in the aim 'the learner will be able to demonstrate basic parenting skills', the teacher acknowledges the need for observable behaviour in the learner.

Consider if any of the following are suitable aims for your antenatal course:

Clients will show they are well prepared for parenthood.
Clients will make the correct health choices for themselves and their babies.
Clients will cope satisfactorily with labour and birth.
Clients will voice and fulfil their needs.
. . . or are your aims something different to the above?

2 Objectives

To be really useful, objectives need to be behavioural, precise, single, realistic and, where possible, measurable. They are behavioural if they are stated in terms of what the client will do, or think, or feel, as a result of your teaching. It is easier to fulfil a precise objective than a vague one. It can be confusing if you try to state objectives in the plural. If you are realistic you are more likely to achieve your objectives. Some objectives, especially those involving exploration of emotions, may be difficult to measure but may nevertheless be of value to the client.

There are different types of objectives:

Cognitive – those to do with gaining knowledge and development of concepts.
Affective – those to do with attitude change or emotions.
Psychomotor – those to do with the acquisition of skills.[3]

Some objectives may contain aspects of more than one type. Awareness of these factors can assist in clarifying what you are attempting to do. You can see how this works if you think about developing appropriate objectives for three common subjects in antenatal education.

(a) DIET IN PREGNANCY

Consider the objective: 'At the end of the session the client will choose a healthy diet.' This objective is cognitive, she must know what constitutes a healthy diet before she can choose one. There may be affective elements, she may need to change her beliefs about 'healthy' food. It is precise, it is single, it is behavioural; she has to do something. Is it measurable? How will you know whether or not she is choosing a healthy diet? Is it realistic? A completely healthy diet may not be feasible if your client is a single mother on a low income, whose educational standard is low, and who is living in bed and breakfast accommodation. Would it be more realistic and measurable to state the objective as: 'My client will recall the constituents of a healthy diet. My client will demonstrate a willingness to adapt her diet within the means at her disposal.'

Antenatal Education Goals

(b) SELF-HELP METHODS OF COPING WITH PAIN IN LABOUR

Consider the objective: 'The client will use the techniques learnt to minimize the pain of labour contractions.' This has psychomotor and cognitive elements. You are teaching skills and she needs to know how and why these techniques work. This objective is behavioural, precise, single and, as stated, it will be measurable when she is in labour. It would be useful, however, to have some assessment of whether or not she has learned the techniques, before she needs to put them into practice. So the objective may be more relevantly stated as: 'My client will recall the techniques she can use during labour to minimize the pain of her contractions.'

Feelings can also affect the way a mother copes with labour, and you may wish to try to change attitudes to pain in labour. Attitude change is often difficult to achieve and to measure. The objective 'My clients will demonstrate a lack of fear about pain in labour' is unrealistic, but an objective such as 'My clients will discuss their hopes and fears for labour' can allow these feelings to be aired and may lead to the desired attitude change.

(c) BABY CARE

Think about the objective: 'At the end of the course the client will care adequately for her baby.' This could be more precise, baby care is a large subject, you need to decide what aspects you wish to cover. She needs knowledge and skills if this objective is to be achieved, but is it realistic to expect her to learn those skills before she has given birth? This objective could be revised to: 'My client will recall a baby's basic needs.' 'My client will demonstrate confidence in her ability to care adequately for her baby.'

Whether or not you agree with these ideas as suitable objectives for antenatal education is not important. What has

Antenatal Education Goals

been demonstrated is, that by attempting to make your objectives precise, realistic and measurable, you are compelled to think clearly about what you are doing, how you are going to do it and how you will know when you have done it. Do not attempt to achieve the perfect set of objectives. If you attempt to be completely realistic, you may run the risk of setting your sights too low. If you are too precise, your objectives may become too narrow and inflexible. If you attempt to teach only that which can be measured, you may deny clients the opportunity to explore their feelings, which can be a valuable learning experience. While formulating your aims and objectives it is useful to bear in mind whether the aims and objectives you set are compatible with what the clients want (see page 26). Also, if the aims and objectives are achieved, consider if the learning that results will be of use to the clients.

3 Assessment

Assessment is linked closely to aims and objectives. Carefully thought-out objectives will often suggest the means of assessment. If you want clients to explore their fears and feelings about pregnancy, a discussion will both fulfil the objective and provide the means to assess it. Discussion in class can allow a client to demonstratre her knowledge of many subjects, as can demonstration of practical skills such as breathing techniques.

Asking questions can stimulate feedback from the clients, but the type of questions you use will affect the quality of that feedback. If you pose an open question, giving enough clues about the information required, and encouragement and opportunity for a full answer, assessment will be possible. A closed question is unlikely to produce a full enough answer and a biased question is likely to receive the answer they think you want (see page 19).

Written work may be appropriate with some groups. Questionnaires or worksheets can be both a learning tool and a

Antenatal Education Goals

form of assessment, and can also be a reminder for clients to retain.

Subjects which may be considered suitable for questionnaires are:

Diet in pregnancy and during breastfeeding.
Choices of pain relief in labour.
Problems with infant feeding.
Illness in babies – when to call the doctor.

Although such questionnaires have a serious intent, they need to be presented in a fairly lighthearted way so that they are not seen as a threat. It is more appropriate if they are like a quiz clients may complete in a woman's magazine rather than school exams.

Assessment of class learning is of limited value without parallel assessment of how that learning is being put to practical use. Access to your clients postnatally is vital if you are to evaluate your work. If you are able to observe some clients in labour, this is advantageous. Liaison with both labour ward staff and clients shortly after delivery is one means of assessing how much knowledge was retained. A questionnaire could be used, either to be completed by the client alone or by client and teacher in the form of a structured interview. Assessment in this situation is of necessity informal, but research programmes are sometimes carried out to attempt a more formal and objective assessment of knowledge gains.[4]

DESIGNING A QUESTIONNAIRE

Keep it short. Clients are unlikely to bother to complete a lengthy questionnaire. Keep it simple. If questions are brief and unambiguous you are more likely to get valid answers. Give clear instructions about how to answer the questions and allow for 'don't knows'. As to layout, leave space, especially between open-ended questions.

Antenatal Education Goals

Ensure anonymity; this will allow for answers which may imply criticism of the teacher. With regard to a particular subject, ask the general questions before the specific. Avoid medical jargon, emotive words and leading questions.

A SAMPLE QUESTIONNAIRE

Sick babies – when to call the doctor

I would call the doctor if:
1. Baby vomited:
   (a) once; (b) twice in one day; (c) all feeds in one day.
2. Baby's stools were:
   (a) green and soft once; (b) green and hard after four days without defaecation; (c) very watery all day.
3. Baby had a rash resulting in:
   (a) red buttocks; (b) three purulent spots in the axilla; (c) red spots all over.
4. Baby's eyes were:
   (a) watery; (b) producing yellow discharge; (c) stuck together in the morning.
5. Baby had a temperature of 37.3°C:
   (a) only if ill; (b) if having convulsions; (c) not if a hot day.
6. Baby fell and hit head:
   (a) always; (b) if unconscious; (c) if floppy and abnormally quiet.
7. Baby cries:
   (a) more than usual; (b) less than usual; (c) differently.
8. Baby haemorrhaged:
   (a) only if severe; (b) if site of origin not obvious; (c) always.
9. Baby swallowed something:
   (a) always; (b) if I knew it was poisonous; (c) if baby seemed in pain.

Antenatal Education Goals

Say in which situations you would:
   Telephone for an appointment with the doctor;
   Ask for a house call;
   Take baby to hospital.
If you suspected your partner or baby sitter had hit your baby, what would you do?

Look critically at this questionnaire. Is it clear what the client is expected to do? Would further instructions be useful and if so what? Are the questions unambiguous? If questions are ambiguous, how could you rephrase them? Do you think your clients would understand all the words? If you believe words are not suitable, what alternatives would you use? Would you increase or decrease the number of questions? Are there any questions you feel it would not be helpful to ask and if so why? Would this questionnaire provide you with either a basis for discussion or an assessment of knowledge gains?

A REUNION CLASS

This provides an opportunity for teacher and clients to discuss the classes, the birth and the first weeks of motherhood and can be a useful opportunity for assessment and evaluation. Again, a questionnaire could be used.

Trigger questions for a reunion class discussion:

Was labour better or worse than you expected it to be?
Is there anything about labour or the birth that you wish you had known but didn't?
Is there anything in your care while you were in hospital that you would like to have changed?
Was there anything you learned in the classes that was particularly useful?
Was there anything about the classes you found unhelpful?

Antenatal Education Goals

What has motherhood been like so far?
What do you feel about the state of your body at present?
What have your emotions been like since the baby was born?

Assisting clients to make self-assessment of their experiences can also serve a useful purpose. A client's expectations may not have been met. Disappointment, guilt and resentment may sour the memories, and affect future behaviour, both in her life generally and in a future pregnancy. A realistic discussion can help to resolve such feelings.

4 Evaluation

Why evaluate? If you don't, how will you know if what you are teaching is of use to your clients? How are you going to correct your mistakes? How are you going to build on your successes and how will you know when you need to make changes?

At the end of every session and at the end of the course look at the objectives you set. Have they been fulfilled?[5] If they have, what particular features do you believe contributed to success? If your objectives were not fulfilled, reflect on possible causes. If clients seemed to lack motivation perhaps you should spend more time discovering what they want to know (see page 26). It may be more important for clients to gain self-confidence rather than a large amount of detailed knowledge.

You may only have the time and resources to carry out informal evaluations, but periodic surveys to evaluate effectiveness and client satisfaction can be useful.

Analysis of what is going on in the classroom and of the activities of the participants, their relationships and transactions, are vital in evaluating and understanding the learning processes. Observing other teachers at work, not necessarily those working within your own discipline, can be helpful in

Antenatal Education Goals

developing this skill. When you understand the types of activities and non-activities which happen in a learning situation – which are likely to aid and which are liable to hinder learning – you will be more able to monitor your own teaching ability. If you have a trusted colleague who understands the value of analysis, you may find it useful to ask her, or him, to observe you. Some observations which are useful are as follows:

Look at the proportion of teacher activity to learner activity. Remember that while the teacher is active, the learners most probably are not.
You need to look at the teacher's attitude to learners and their efforts. An accepting attitude is helpful, a critical attitude is not normally helpful.
Both learner-to-learner and teacher-to-learner interaction needs to take place for maximum learning.
Reflect whether the teacher really listens to what the learners say.
Learners who look bored are probably not learning.
Look at the body language of teacher and learners. Assertion and openness are positive factors, aggression and submission are negative factors.
Consider whether the teacher demonstrates awareness of the non-verbal messages coming from the learners. For example, hunched posture and lack of eye contact from a learner may show either a lack of desire or an inability to participate in the session.
Using the learners' names is one way of recognising their individuality and worth.
Once you are aware of the significance of both verbal and non-verbal activities you can use them to review and develop your teaching.[6,7]

It is not easy to assess and evaluate antenatal education, but both objective and subjective feedback can be used. A client may feel the classes have helped her to cope with the stress of labour and her subjective evaluation should be regarded as important as a more objective measurement of knowledge gains.

References

1 Black, P. M., Faulkner, A. M., Thompson, A. M. (1984), 'Antenatal classes: a selective review of the literature,' *Nurse Education Today*, vol. 3, no. 6, pp. 130–3.
2 French, J. and Adams, L. (1986), 'From analysis to synthesis. Theories of health education', *Health Education Journal*, vol. 45, no. 2, pp. 71–3.
3 Bloom, B. S. *et al.* (1956), *Taxonomy of Educational Objectives*, Handbook 1: *Cognitive Domain*; (1964) Handbook 2: *Affective Domain*, Longman, London.
4 Husband, L. (1983), 'Antenatal education: Its use and effectiveness', *Health Visitor*, vol. 56, pp. 409–10.
5 Brown, A. (1986), *Groupwork*, Gower, Aldershot, pp. 104–8.
6 Flanders, N. A. (1970), *Analysing Teacher Behaviour*, Addison-Wesley, New York, p. 448.
7 Jacques, D. (1984), *Learning in Groups*, Croom Helm, London, pp. 217–33.

Further Reading

Berne, E. (1964), *Games People Play. The Psychology of Human Relationships*, Penguin, Harmondsworth.
Ewles, L. and Simnett, I. (1985), *Promoting Health. A Practical Guide to Health Education*, John Wiley & Sons, Chichester.
Fast, J. (1971), *Body Language*, Pan, London.
Hibbard, B. M., Robinson, J. O., Pearson, J. F., Rosen, M. and Taylor, A. (1979), 'The effectiveness of antenatal education', *Health Education Journal*, vol. 38, no. 2, pp. 39–46.
Murphy-Black, T. and Faulkner, A. (1988), *Antenatal Group Skills Training. A Manual of Guidelines*, John Wiley & Sons, Chichester.
Perkins, E. R. (1979), Defining the need: an analysis of varying goals in antenatal classes', *International Journal of Nursing Studies*, vol. 16, pp. 275–82.

2
Theories of Learning

Learning is an essential human activity. We may learn consciously or unconsciously, but we have to learn if we are to survive. Learning involves change in an individual which will subsequently affect behaviour. When we learn we take in information, try to make sense of that information in the light of previous learning and experience, see the relevance of that information to ourselves and assimilate the knowledge. Then we make the changes that seem appropriate; these changes may be in behaviour, or attitude, or both.

1 Motivation

Consider what makes people want to learn. Motivation is the spur that drives us to satisfy a need or achieve a goal. Needs can be basic survival needs: we need to learn how to satisfy our hunger, to stay warm and safe, to earn a living. We also seek to satisfy our desire to know about what interests us, to learn how to be accepted by others, to be loved or belong to a group. We also seek to find fulfilment in our lives, to be happy.[1] Given the opportunity, people will learn what they want to learn or what they believe they need to learn. However, there are many influences, including psychological and cultural, which affect how people perceive their needs. What is important to antenatal teachers is that people will not learn what they do not want to learn or what they do not believe is useful for them (see page 17). They will either not attend classes or just 'switch off'. For example, a mother may expect a normal birth. She therefore sees no need to learn about forceps delivery or Caesarean birth. Even if this is taught she will probably not retain the information. Where there is no perceived need, learning is unlikely to take place.

2 How We Learn

Many educationalists and psychologists have studied how both animals and humans learn.[2] Various theories of learning have been developed and there are two which have important implications for antenatal teachers – conditioning and trial and error.

(a) CONDITIONING

One way in which we learn is described by educational theorists as 'operant conditioning'. In this the learner receives a stimulus and makes a response, which in turn produces a result. If the result is pleasant or productive the response is likely to be repeated; if the result is unpleasant or unproductive it is not likely to be repeated when the stimulus is received again. For example, think of a child learning to cross a busy road safely. If the child's response is to dash across without care, the result may be that he is frightened and his mother is angry – an unpleasant result. If his response is to follow the safety code, the result is more likely to be a happy and satisfactory experience which will be repeated more readily. Conditioning continues through life, as we respond to various stimuli.

Previous conditioning can affect the way we approach a learning situation. Faced with an antenatal class in a room furnished with chairs in rows and with a teacher who stands in front of a blackboard, how do you think a mother who hated school, failed all her exams and resents authority will react? She has been conditioned by her previous experiences, she has

Theories of Learning

learned that school meant fear, failure and misery. Any situation that is similar is likely to evoke that conditioning and therefore learning is unlikely to take place. Previous conditioning can be overcome but the teacher needs to be sure that she is not inadvertently reinforcing what she is attempting to change. For example, although attitudes are beginning to change there is still the feeling in society that childbirth is always painful, is meant to be painful and there is nothing the mother can do about it herself. The antenatal teacher might say 'Birth can be a joyful experience, you have resources within yourself to cope with and minimize the pain.' But her attitude might say, 'You are correct to believe that unbearable pain is part of giving birth to your baby, you will need to rely on us to relieve that pain.' It is more likely the message conveyed by the attitude will be received by the client, because it reinforces her previous learning. Knowledge and attitudes are both learned and can be reinforced or changed by subsequent learning.

(b) TRIAL AND ERROR LEARNING

This can occur when there is opportunity for a learner to attempt many different solutions to a problem. In a 'trial and error' educational situation, the teacher will set up the problem and then leave the learners to work without guidance. While excellent results can be obtained from this type of teaching, it is time-consuming and difficult to apply in a pure form to antenatal teaching. Your clients cannot solve, by actual trial and error, the problem of what method of pain relief will be best for them in labour. What you can do is to set before them the available information and ask them to consider the 'pros' and 'cons'.

Setting up a problem-solving situation will encourage the learners to be active (see page 18). Where possible the teacher should allow the students to work through the problem with the minimum of interference, because the more active the

Theories of Learning

teacher the less active the student.

Much parenting is trial and error. By encouraging your clients to consider problems and how to attempt to solve them, you will enable them to discover resources which will help them later. A problem-solving approach to learning helps to foster confidence and self-reliance in a client rather than dependence on a teacher.

3 Factors That Affect Learning

(a) PREVIOUS LEARNING

We all try to make sense of our world, but we can do this only in the light of our previous experiences. It may be impossible to make sense of information presented to us if it does not relate to something we already know. For example, we need basic numeracy skills before we can study higher mathematics. This applies not only to the cognitive domain but also to the affective domain. For example, a client whose own mothering experience was of an unloving, uncaring, unresponsive person, may find it difficult to understand the concept of bonding between mother and baby.

You need to think about the knowledge base of your clients. Learning about the physiology of labour may be impossible, however well and simply explained, if you assume a basic knowledge of anatomy your clients do not possess. Think about whether you use an appropriate language level. Medical terms and other words less frequently used in general conversation may not be understood by everyone. The way the words are put together is also important. Short simple sentences may be more appropriate than ones that are long and complicated. It can sometimes be difficult to pitch the level just right in a mixed group. 'Talking down' to learners can be as counterproductive to learning as using long words they don't understand. Metaphors are one way of communicating concepts but

Theories of Learning

are only useful if the images used are familiar. If you use 'waves on the sea' to describe the sensation of labour contractions, you need to ask yourself if any of your clients come from countries where they had no experience of the sea and for whom this image has no meaning.

(b) PERCEPTION

Each individual's previous learning and therefore her perception of the world is unique. A group of people may all *see* (or hear or smell or taste or feel) the same thing but may all *perceive* something different.[3]

A word can have many meanings and interpretations.[4] These evolve as a result of many influences – culture, education and life experiences – and are therefore unique to each individual.[5] A teacher should try to be aware of the learner's understanding of the words used and may need to clarify her own definition of the words she is using. Consider 'normal birth' and 'natural birth'. Some people would equate the two phrases, others would apply 'natural' only to a labour free of all drugs and medical intervention. A midwife would record a birth as 'normal' if she had delivered the baby with the aid of an episiotomy; others may consider this to be medical intervention and therefore not 'normal'.

(c) RELEVANCE

Significant learning will not take place if an individual perceives the information as having no relevance to herself.[6] Information remembered and understood, but with no perceived relevance, will therefore have no effect on attitude or behaviour and cannot be said to be truly learned. Consider how many smokers remember and understand the anti-smoking information but continue to smoke.

Theories of Learning

(d) MEMORY

Although learning is more than remembering facts, memory is important.[7] Repetition aids memory, so allow time for this in your teaching. If too much information is presented at one time or presented in a dull fashion, it may be difficult to remember. We can all recall a boring lecture in which the information 'went in one ear and out of the other'.

(e) ACTIVITY

Can knowledge be handed from one person to another like the giving of a gift, or forced upon an individual like a mother bird stuffing food down the throat of a nestling? No, true learning demands activity on the part of the learner.

Do we learn by listening, by watching or by doing? Think about skills you have acquired. Can you knit? Can you swim? Do you drive a car or play the piano? What about your midwifery skills, delivering a baby, giving an injection, estimating cervical dilatation? We may need some instruction and demonstration, but the most important factor is practice. However hesitantly, however inefficiently we do it at first, we have to *do* it. The same principle can be applied to learning that does not involve physical action. Judgemental skills are also needed in midwifery. As students we do not automatically learn how to care for a woman in labour merely because we have been told. We receive instruction, we observe qualified midwives and then we practise under supervision. Gradually we become more skilled at making judgements about the care of our clients as we practise making those judgements. Think back again to that boring lecture. Was any part of you active? You were sitting still, but what about your brain? Was it active? Now try to recall a lesson at school or during your training, one in which the knowledge really stuck. Almost certainly the teacher arranged that session so that you had to think, so that your brain or body was active.

Theories of Learning

Some of the subjects we teach involve physical skills, like bathing a baby, or relaxation. But much of what we try to teach is concerned with mothers learning to make decisions and judgements. Each mother has to decide what she should eat when she is pregnant, whether to have pain relief in labour, and if so what she should have. She also will learn to judge what her baby's needs are when he cries. If teaching situations are structured to encourage activity on the part of the learner rather than merely presenting them with information, more true learning is likely to result. Is this book giving you answers or is it making you think? Is it making you reflect on what you already know, encouraging you to try out ideas to discover for yourself what is useful, stimulating you to seek out further knowledge? If it is making you think, then it is achieving its objective. If it is giving you answers, then it has failed. The concept of learning from and through experience is one that deserves serious consideration by all teachers.[8]

One way of encouraging learner activity is by asking questions, but what type of questions best serve this purpose? Questions which require only a one-word answer and which do not make clients think are unlikely to stimulate activity.

For example, 'Have you bought a pram?' This is a closed question: the obvious answer is 'yes' or 'no' and it provides little stimulation for further discussion.

'How is the baby going to travel around after it is born?' This question is too open, too vague, leaving the client uncertain as to what is expected in reply.

'Newborn babies look so exposed and vulnerable in buggies, is anyone planning to use one?' A biased question which is more likely to be answered in agreement with the bias.

'Have you decided on a pram yet; do you think a buggy or pram is best, of course you need to consider the safety factors; do you know about the British Standards Institution?' A multiple question which is confusing and difficult to remember.

Now consider the question: 'Many mothers are now buying

Theories of Learning

a 'lie back' buggy rather than a larger pram for their newborn babies. What advantages or disadvantages do you think this has?' You have given them some information to consider: your question requires them to give an opinion, to make a judgement based on what knowledge they have. Different clients are likely to give different answers, thus stimulating discussion. That discussion allows a pooling of knowledge, opens the possibility of sharing a wider range of opinions and allows misinformation to be corrected.

(f) REWARDS AND PUNISHMENTS

These often play a part in children's education and much of the research into the effects has validity for all learners. Punishment obviously has no place in antenatal education, although there can sometimes be subtle punishment in the form of teacher disapproval. Some understanding of the psychological effects of rewards can be useful.[9]

Rewards can be extrinsic – coming from outside the learner, awarded by the teacher – or intrinsic – originating from within the student, the satisfaction the learner has with her own efforts. Obvious extrinsic rewards are high exam marks, prizes or gold stars; not so obvious but also extrinsic is praise from a teacher or even approval of, for example, a client's decision to breastfeed her baby. Extrinsic rewards may cause learners to seek a correct answer rather than trying to find a way to solve a problem. This has limited value. A 'correct' answer can be achieved by client without learning having taken place. For example, the question 'How do you plan to feed your baby?' may elicit the answer 'Breastfeed.' The client having picked up clues from the teacher which indicates this is what the teacher sees as desirable, that is the *correct* answer. If, however, the learner is directed towards problem solving, she may be encouraged to consider all aspects of baby feeding and make the decision she believes is correct for her. Learning through problem solving leads to greater intrinsic

Theories of Learning

rewards. If an individual feels inner satisfaction with her efforts she is more likely to continue to try to learn more.

(g) TEACHER/LEARNER RELATIONSHIPS

How are you perceived by your clients?

As the remote professional.
As the expert who has all the answers.
As the knowledgeable but approachable person of whom they can ask anything.
As the person who values them as people and is there to help them learn what they want to know.

More significant learning is likely to take place if the learner believes herself to be valued as a person. This is known as 'unconditional positive regard'.[10]

How do we perceive them? And, what is probably more important, how do they believe we perceive them?

As people ignorant of the subjects being taught.
As people full of misconceptions to be corrected.
As people who need to be taught what is good for them.
As people who have needs to be catered for.
As people who have the right and responsibility to take control of their own lives.

We should consider the accuracy of our perceptions of our clients.

Are they ignorant?
Did they study biology at school?
Have mother, sister and/or friend talked of birth experiences?
Have they young siblings, sister or friend with young children or is this a second pregnancy?
Do they watch television or read?

Theories of Learning

They may have absorbed some inaccurate knowledge which needs correcting, but is the way we see things necessarily 100 per cent correct? Do we know what is good for them? Are the medical professions the ultimate guardians of health?[11] Will clients first have to discover and then learn how to voice their needs. Are we free to allow them to discover their real needs? Those in positions of power or authority may have vested interests that prevent this happening.[12] Do clients need encouragement to take responsibility for themselves?

How we perceive them will affect the way we teach them, and how they believe we perceive them will affect the way they learn. There is a tendency for people to live up to others' expectations of them. Have you ever experienced a situation where you found it difficult to grasp something that you were being taught, maybe compounded by the fact that everyone else seemed to understand and you felt the teacher thought you were stupid? If you have no such memory, imagine how you would feel. Would you be happy to keep on trying until you did understand, or would you feel threatened, anxious, even panic-stricken – as stupid as you believed the teacher thought you were? How do you feel if someone criticizes you, or regards your opinions as valueless? Happy? Eager to learn from them? How do you react when someone tries to force you to do something that is 'good for you'?

Think of a teacher you liked, someone you thought was a good teacher, from whom you found it easy to learn. Or think of a friend or colleague whose opinions you valued. How did that person treat you? People learn best when they feel unthreatened, safe to make mistakes and when they feel the teacher regards them as worthwhile individuals. If that regard is not genuine it will be detected. Does this mean that to be a good teacher one has to be a paragon of all the virtues? Of course not, but if your clients see you as a real person, not playing a role or putting up a façade, as someone who accepts them for what they are, not judging them and with ability to empathize and show congruence,[13] then they are more likely

Theories of Learning

to learn. 'Accepting' behaviour in a teacher may include self-disclosure. It can be appropriate to use personal experiences or admit to feelings a client may be reluctant to reveal. For example, 'I was apprehensive/frightened when I began labour.' However, care should be taken not to endorse undesirable behaviour.[14]

Your own feelings as a teacher also deserve consideration. As a new teacher do you feel anxious, threatened, frightened of making a fool of yourself? Wouldn't it be more comfortable if you did play the role of *teacher*, the professional. A façade means you don't have to expose *yourself*. Many new antenatal teachers feel reluctant because they feel unprepared for the job they have undertaken. Uncertainty is unnerving, but if we can see the problems and challenges as part of an ongoing process of learning to teach, rather than a threat to our sense of personal worth, we will experience less fear and apprehension.

None of us is perfect. Don't be afraid to admit there are things you do not know, though you are willing to find out. Don't be disheartened when you have a disappointing session; it happens to the most experienced teachers. Do be prepared to learn from both the good and bad experiences. Don't be afraid to let your clients know you as a real person; it will be more rewarding for them and you. Don't forget, although you have a responsibility to equip yourself as thoroughly as possible, the ultimate responsibility for learning lies with the learners. You cannot force them to learn.

References

1. Child, D. (1981), *Psychology and the Teacher*, Holt, Rhinehart and Winston, London, pp. 33–64.
2. *Ibid.*, pp. 81–111.
3. Abercrombie, M. L. J. (1960), *The Anatomy of Judgement. An Investigation into the Processes of Perception and Reasoning*, Penguin, Harmondsworth, pp. 25–76.

4   *Ibid.*, pp. 110–31.
5   Postman, N. and Weingartner, C. (1969), *Teaching as a Subversive Activity*, Penguin, Harmondsworth, pp. 100–27.
6   *Ibid.*, p. 59.
7   Child, *Psychology and the Teacher*, pp. 112–34.
8   Burnard, P. (1985), *Learning Human Skills. A Guide for Nurses*, Heinemann, London, pp. 29–55.
9   Child, *Psychology and the Teacher*.
10 Rogers, C. R. (1961), *On Becoming a Person. A Therapist's View of Psychotherapy*, Constable, London, pp. 283–4.
11 Illich, I. (1976), 'Limits to medicine,' *Medical Nemesis: The Expropriation of Health*, Penguin, Harmondsworth.
12 Postman and Weingartner, *Teaching as a Subversive Activity*, pp. 15–27.
13 Rogers, *On Becoming a Person*, pp. 61–2, 282–3, 339–42.
14 Brown, A. (1986), Groupwork, Gower, Aldershot, pp. 66–9.

Further Reading

Borger, R. and Seaborne, A. E. M. (1982), *The Psychology of Learning*, 2nd edn, Penguin, Harmondsworth.

Holt, J. (1982), *How Children Fail*, 2nd edn, Penguin, Harmondsworth.

3

Planning

To become a confident, competent teacher you need to plan your work carefully and thoroughly. After you have formulated your aims and objectives, ensure you have a thorough knowledge of your subjects. Enthusiasm for what you are doing is an asset. You should also seek to discover your clients' particular needs. Teaching methods and aids should be appropriate to the subject and client group. Many antenatal teachers do not work in isolation and using expertise from many disciplines can be a valuable resource.

1 Subject Knowledge

(a) DO YOU KNOW YOUR SUBJECT?

Are you insulted by that question? Please don't be. Midwifery training may not prepare you for all the questions mothers ask. You may have to consider some subjects for the first time or in greater depth or from a different viewpoint. For example, evaluation of safety and efficiency in the design of baby equipment is not normally taught in midwifery training schools. Continuing progress in midwifery and obstetrics demands frequent updating. Wide media coverage of medical advances can mean that clients possess some knowledge of those advances and these need explanation or interpretation. Awareness of the media will alert you to the issues clients may raise. Professional journals can help to keep you up to date. Some suggestions for resources are made at the end of this chapter.

Planning

(b) DO YOU BELIEVE IN WHAT YOU ARE DOING?

Can you think of a teacher who was enthusiastic about his subject, or a friend who was enthusiastic about a hobby, or a film she had seen? So that you wanted to learn, or try out that hobby or see the film? If you show a real interest in what you are teaching, the clients are more likely to want to learn. A teacher who is bored with a subject is likely to convey that boredom to the learners. But beware, over-enthusiasm can also produce boredom. Do you like to learn? The best teachers are perpetual learners.

2 Client Need

(a) DISCOVERING CLIENT NEED

When clients are asked, they agree the subjects most commonly discussed in antenatal classes are useful to them. Interest is shown in well-being in pregnancy, fetal development, labour, birth and infant care, but somewhat less interest in what clients perceive as the abnormal aspects such such as fetal monitoring and Caesarean sections.[1] Antenatal classes have not always lived up to expectations and although some were considered realistic in their preparation of mothers, help in the practical and emotional factors of childcare was not felt to be adequate.[2-4] This is borne out by one study which showed that mothers were ill-prepared for parenthood.[5] Reading material is often quoted as an important source of information.[6,7,8] Given that in classes only a limited part of the information presented will be remembered, providing leaflets, and possibly a library, can be a useful back-up to your teaching.

Clients are individuals and will have different needs. You need to think about how you can discover those needs. We should be wary of stereotyping, but it can be helpful to know

Planning

something of clients' backgrounds. Knowing the area in which they live, their educational level, their cultural background, their age and parity can be useful information to help us assess their needs. Some information you can obtain from patient records, some simply from being aware of the area in which you are working, some from meeting them and hearing them speak. Such information can prepare you for their possible expectations, cultural taboos or requirements of behaviour.

Consider asking your clients what they wish to learn. Clients may be more receptive to your teaching if the programme has been negotiated with them. You will probably teach the same subjects, but the emphasis, order and timing may vary with each group. Timing is important, your audience may be more or less receptive to learning about a subject according to the stage of pregnancy reached. For example, consider when you should teach baby care. It may seem too distant and therefore irrelevant early in pregnancy, but late in pregnancy their minds may be preoccupied with thoughts of labour. Sensitivity to each group will allow you to choose the appropriate time for teaching particular subjects. As your relationship with each group develops, some needs will become apparent. As they discover their own needs and accept and trust you, they will be more able to voice them.

Several research studies highlight the importance mothers placed on the social contact with other mothers at antenatal classes,[9,10,11] Provision for this, for example a refreshment break which allows time for chat, can facilitate friendships and mutual support.

(b) ATTENDANCE AT CLASSES

We cannot teach clients if they do not attend. How do we ensure they come? First, think about how they are invited. Notices may be insufficient; a personal invitation whether verbal or written is more likely to be accepted.[12,13] If clients are invited at the booking visit and the classes do not start until

Planning

weeks later, a reminder may be necessary at a later clinic visit. If professionals demonstrate enthusiasms and skill, putting a value on antenatal education, clients are more likely to take antenatal education seriously.[14,15,16] You would do well to consider the reasons clients have given for non-attendance; inconvenient location, difficulties with transport, inconvenient times, clashing with work or family commitments, lack of crèche facilities.[17,18,19,20] It may not be within your power to alter your classes to suit everyone, but think if you could make any useful changes. Perceiving classes as not relevant or useful is another reason given. Making the classes interesting and relevant is important, but give some thought to whether your classes are offered in a way that will attract the clients.[21]

(c) A BROADER VIEW OF HEALTH NEEDS

We can think of specific client need in the antenatal situation, but if we take a broader view, we can consider how our teaching could have a far-reaching influence on health (see Chapter 1). Clients attending antenatal classes may have a clear idea of their immediate learning needs. You can also help them to discover other unspoken or unrealized needs. Although economic and political influences mean that many individuals probably never will have complete control of the determinants of their health, you can assist them to learn that their health is largely within their own power to control.[22] It is a right and a responsibility you can encourage them to exercise. You can do this even without raising any major issues for discussion, if the way you teach is acknowledging the validity of their opinions, encouraging them to make decisions for themselves instead of merely accepting what is done to them. 'The medium is the message'.[23]

(d) PLANNING FOR SPECIAL NEEDS

Clients with particular needs may present on a regular basis;

Planning

clients with a poor understanding of English are one example. Careful attention to the words you use and clear, appropriate visual aids will be helpful. If you have only an occasional client with a language problem, you could invite her to bring an interpreter. If you are working with a wholly immigrant group, can you obtain and work through an interpreter? Can you use the classes to help them improve their English?[24]

Clients with blindness, deafness and various physical disabilities may need your special attention. Frequently other agencies, for example the Royal National Institute for the Blind or the Disabled Living Foundation, will be involved in helping these women prepare for parenthood (see Appendix 1). With forethought these clients can often benefit from participating in a group. Tactile aids for the blind and a basic knowledge of sign language can aid the deaf.[25]

Teenagers may not attend because they do not feel the regular classes relate to their needs. A teenage group which is designed specifically to cater for their requirements and organized on a more informal 'club' basis can become a successful support resource for young mothers.[26,27,28]

Adoptive parents have need of only part of the usual antenatal classes but are often a neglected group. They obviously need child-care information but the emotional adjustment they have to make is often forgotten.[29] They may or may not wish to join pregnant couples and a special group may be able to fulfil their needs.[30]

Mothers who have suffered an interuterine death will probably find it too stressful to attend a group and may need one-to-one sessions.

3 Teaching Methods

Successful teaching requires a variety of methods and changes of pace, often within one session. Every method of teaching requires skill from the teacher and co-operation from the

Planning

student; boredom is always a possibility. When deciding what method you will use, you need to think about what teacher and learner are doing, consider the advantages and disadvantages, and which method is appropriate to particular subjects and client groups.

(a) LECTURE

Teacher talking, learner listening.

Advantages
It is easy to convey a lot of information quickly, useful to introduce a subject, and when information is not otherwise easily available to learners.

Disadvantages
Lecture time often exceeds attention span, which even in university students, when the maximum span could be expected, may be only twenty minutes. Students are passive, there is no feedback to the teacher and it is not possible to cater for different needs.

While it is to be hoped that a whole antenatal class would not be one long lecture, when you introduce a subject, or present new information, this is a mini-lecture.

(b) DISCUSSION GROUP

Teacher and learners both talking and listening.

Advantages
Students are active and, with practice, their ability to discuss and decide improves. Sharing increases learning, many different viewpoints can be put forward and, consequently, there is greater stimulation. Presenting information for discussion is obviously important, but members of the group could be encouraged to raise points too. Many groups may collectively

Planning

possess a large amount of knowledge which they can be encouraged to share. In discussion you can not only make the dissemination of knowledge easier but also correct misinformation and check learning.

Disadvantages
There may be inequality of participation; some talk too much, some not enough. It takes skill to create a productive discussion. If students are unfamiliar with this method of teaching, they may find it difficult or threatening.

Discussion groups are a popular and useful teaching method of teaching for antenatal classes and are considered in greater detail later.

(c) BUZZ GROUP

Similar to discussion but smaller and shorter.

Advantage
It has the advantages of a discussion group, but with greater informality, and is useful to split large groups. More ground can be covered and it gives more opportunities for all to participate.

Disadvantages
Can be noisy and needs space to split up a large group. The teacher cannot monitor all, but this is not necessarily a disadvantage since a freer discussion sometimes occurs without teacher presence. Some participants may feel increased pressure to contribute. If one is shy it is easier to hide in a large group.

(d) TRIAL AND ERROR, PROBLEM SOLVING

Teacher sets up the problem, learners work with or without guidance.

Advantages
Students are active and there is good retention of knowledge. The significance of that knowledge is greater because it is self-discovered.[31] It can be used with an individual or group.

Disadvantages
Needs skill to plan and time to execute. If learners are truly to learn by this method they must be allowed to work at their own pace.

(e) DEMONSTRATION

Teacher demonstrates, learners watch.

Advantages
Useful where the information is more easily conveyed visually.

Disadvantages
Students are passive. The number able to observe may be limited.

(f) PRACTICAL SESSION

Teacher supervises, learners work.

Advantages
Students are active, activity aids memory and understanding. Combined with demonstration is an efficient way of acquiring a skill.

Disadvantages
Need space and equipment in quantity, and the availability of these commodities may limit the number of participants. Teacher may not be able to monitor all the learners.

Planning

(g) ROLE PLAY

Teacher sets up situation, learners act out, followed by discussion of what was experienced.[32,33]

Advantages
Students are active. Feelings as well as intellect are used, so helping clients to relate the situation portrayed to their own lives. Can be fun, putting over a serious point in a lighthearted way.

Disadvantages
Needs skill and time to prepare. The teacher needs to be aware of the various directions the role play could take, being prepared to cope with a situation that becomes too distressing for the participants. Inhibitions can prevent participation. It is open to misinterpretation. It may be threatening and participation should never be forced. Time must be allowed for 'de-briefing', giving opportunity for coming to terms with any negative feelings.

(h) VISITS

Teacher and learners visiting relative venue.

Advantages
Usually an enjoyable activity for learners. Can inject reality when the learning situation is new and the information unfamiliar. May make available more material than could be presented in class.

Disadvantages
This is time-consuming and needs careful organization. There is a danger it may be just entertaining with no real educational value.

Planning

(i) ONE-TO-ONE

Teacher and learner working together, either can be active.

Advantages
It is possible to cater for individual needs. This can take place on a planned basis or as and when the need arises. It is flexible, can be information giving, discussion or demonstration/practical session.

Disadvantages
It is time-consuming. Relationship problems can be magnified with intimacy, a clash of personalities can make learning difficult or client may come to use the teacher in an inappropriate way as an emotional prop.

4 Group Work

(a) PLANNING

The size of a group influences behaviour and what activities can be undertaken. For example, a larger group can be divided into sub-groups, to work on different aspects of a subject before joining together in a plenary session.[34] You may have no control over the number in your group, but the type of activities and relationships sought by antenatal teachers works well with a group of between eight to twelve. In groups larger than fifteen it is more difficult to foster the close personal relationships which can add to the clients' satisfaction. Discussions are possible in larger groups. Splitting a large group into smaller buzz groups for short periods before a plenary session can also work well.

A pleasant venue can aid group work. Look at the room in which you will teach. Is the atmosphere and layout conducive to a relaxed and open discussion? Providing comfortable

Planning

chairs or flowers and pretty curtains may not be within your control, but think what you could do to make your venue more welcoming. Colourful posters are a simple way of brightening a drab room. It is more difficult to have a good discussion in a classroom atmosphere. Probably the most important consideration is the seating. Seating, either chairs, beanbags or foam wedges, in a circle will allow everyone to have eye contact with each other, which will aid discussion better than chairs in rows. A circle means that there is no obvious 'teacher' position, allowing the teacher to function as a member of the group. If you do not wear a uniform, this can also help. It is helpful if the teacher is on the same physical level as the students rather than above them.[35]

As with any teaching session you will need to think out your aims and objectives. In group work, there may be more aims and objectives that are to do with feelings and attitudes. These objectives are often more difficult to assess, and the teacher may have to be content with the discussion itself as an objective, rather than any measurable change. One can only hope the discussion will stimulate further thought and the desired change may come later.

In group work it is well to bear in mind that flexibility is advantageous. Be prepared to sacrifice some specific objectives in a session if by doing so you allow them to fulfil another objective or one of the more general aims of the course. For example, if they fail to discuss all the pros and cons of breast- and bottlefeeding and instead have a deep discussion about personal responsibility in decision making in health, that may be of equal or greater value to your clients.

(b) LEADERSHIP STYLE

The style of leadership will affect the quality and quantity of learning within the group. An autocratic leader who keeps strict control of the group may enable learners to achieve a greater number of tasks but may produce dependence and

Planning

possibly resentment. A democratic leader who makes decisions about subjects and activities in co-operation with group members is likely to achieve a good amount of learning, with greater learner satisfaction. Learners who receive very little direction from a leader may achieve less. No one style of leadership is correct for every group, indeed a leader may employ different styles with one group at different times, being sensitive to the productive and non-productive interactions taking place.[36]

(c) FACILITATING DISCUSSION

Getting started
There are several strategies that can be employed to encourage strangers to talk to one another. Some sort of naming or other introductory activity can be used:

1   Each member in turn is asked to introduce themselves by name and give one fact about themselves, e.g. 'My name is Jane and this is my first baby.'
2   Clients are asked to talk in pairs, then introduce each other.
3   First person says her own name, second person says the first name then her own name, third person says the first and second names, then her own name etc. until the last person says all the names of the group.
4   Each member is asked in turn for some comment, such as 'What I like/don't like about being pregnant is . . .', 'What I want from the classes is . . .' or possibly something unconnected with the situation, such as 'What I had for breakfast this morning', or 'I had a good/bad journey here today because . . .'

This activity needs to be non-threatening and can be started with a comment from the teacher. It must be made clear that participation is voluntary. What you judge to be a non-threatening situation may be a dreadful ordeal to a client.

Planning

Getting started on the subject

Some sort of introduction is necessary, it can be a short talk by the teacher, a trigger film or just one well chosen question (see page 19). Recognize that you are expecting people to interact with you and each other. Every member of the group will have her own attitudes, feelings and 'hang ups'. Everyone, except the very socially deprived, has discussions in their daily lives, even if it is only about the latest TV soap opera. Many, however, may feel shy and threatened when asked to discuss matters in a slightly more formal way. It takes time for each member to work out her relationships with the other members, to decide what she is trying to get out of the discussions and what she can give.

Keeping going

There will be changes in the way the group reacts, especially if the same group of people are together over a period of time. There will be a time of discovery, a time to get to know the leader, each other and what they are there for, a time for exploring possibilities.

Eventually the group must get to grips with the task in hand. Sometimes they may argue, sometimes co-operate, sometimes disagree with the leader, sometimes seek leadership. Leadership may come from one other than the appointed. If the message is correct, do you always have to be seen to be in charge? If the group is following the direction or reaching conclusions which are desirable, who the apparent leader is at any one time is not important. Support for a diffident member or a request for clarification can come from any member. Group cohesiveness will be enhanced as more interactions of this type occur. In a dynamic group different people at different times may play the various roles: leader, supporter, stimulator, clarifier, summarizer. The role of the appointed leader is that of facilitator, 'helping things happen'. You can plan beforehand the strategies to employ, but during the session be constantly aware of all the non-verbal clues the

Planning

group members are displaying, and that includes yourself. Is your own body language relaxed and accepting? Eye contact aids discussion, but too much with one individual can be threatening. Look at the clients' behaviour. Is the quiet one showing behaviour that says 'With a little encouragement I could have something to say'? Is the blank look saying 'I am not interested', or maybe, 'I don't understand'?

If someone asks a question, do you have to answer it? You can invite a reply from the group, with a remark such as: 'Does anyone know the answer to that question?' If you ask a question and receive an answer, you can ask the respondent or another to elaborate on the reply. These techniques will facilitate real discussion rather than a question and answer session directed at the teacher. When you ask a question, allow a pause of about five seconds for a reply. If you get no reply, re-phrase the question or try another. If there is still no response, give the clients something more to think about. Do not repeatedly ask questions if you get no response; this becomes interrogation.

Criticism is not normally helpful in this situation. You may need to correct misinformation, but try to do it in a way that does not imply a critical attitude. For example, if a client talks of 'gas and air', instead of saying 'No, that is wrong, it is not gas and air, it is gas and oxygen', you could say, 'We tend to say gas and air, because that is what it used to be, but it has been changed to gas and oxygen, which is important for you and your baby.'

If clients appear uninterested reflect on why this is so. Maybe they just need some fuel: a little more information from you, a visual aid for them to consider, a question to trigger their thoughts (see page 19). They may not see the subject as relevant to themselves, so try to present the subject so that they do see the relevance. The clients' views are valid, and perhaps they don't need to consider a particular subject at the time you present it. Are you flexible and courageous enough to abandon it and go on to something else? Even if you

Planning

believe it is vital for the clients to have some particular information, the session is not likely to be productive if you persist when there is lack of interest. Silences are not necessarily negative. Time for reflection can be useful. It can take courage at first to allow silences, as they tend to be embarrassing, but if you can show by your attitude that you are content to allow this to happen, your students will soon learn to accept them. Observation of the group will tell you if they are embarrassed, bored or thoughtful.

You may have no difficulty in getting them to talk, but they may not stay on the subject that you proposed. Think whether you need to bring them back to the agenda, or whether the subject they are discussing is valid, within your overall plan. If it is something you would be discussing later, you could, with advantage, allow it to continue. They are interested in it *now* and perhaps you will have a better discussion than if you stop them and try to re-introduce the subject at a later date. If you feel it is necessary to change the subject, possible phrases to use are: 'That is interesting but before we talk any more about it, can we first think about . . . or, 'We have talked a little about . . . and I would like us to think about it in more detail next week. Can you tell me what you feel about . . .' If the discussion degenerates into idle chatter, you may need to bring them back to your subject. Humour can be useful here: a heavy-handed approach may stop them talking altogether.

(e) DEALING WITH PROBLEM MEMBERS

The one who talks too much
This can be a problem because it prevents others from contributing. It can also restrict the range of subject matter covered. You need to think about how you will deal with this problem. If this person talks for a long time you may need to interrupt, if possible at a natural break rather than mid-sentence, inviting others to comment on what she has said or to make their own contribution. Or you may thank her for her

Planning

contribution and suggest a change of subject. If she is always the one to respond when a question is asked, try to suggest that it is fairer to let everyone have a chance to talk. When asking a question, avoid catching her eye. Look for a response from someone else. Try not to 'put her down'; this is not only unkind but may upset her so that she stops learning and it can cause an uncomfortable atmosphere which destroys the group cohesiveness. Why is she talking so much? Is she just being selfish, or does she have a need that is not being fulfilled? You may be able to help her in a one-to-one session after the class.

The one who will not talk at all
It is possible she is just a shy person who needs time to get to know the others. If the ambience of the group is friendly and supportive, with gentle encouragement she will probably find her feet eventually. Forcing her, demanding a contribution, will not be helpful. If she is different in some way to the majority (colour, speech, education or age), you can try to play down the differences and emphasize the similarities, thus making her feel one of the group. She may be a person who does not talk much, but does learn from hearing the others talk and that is her privilege.

The one who argues and challenges everything that is said
This person can act as a useful catalyst, stimulating discussion. But if she is too argumentative, this can prove disruptive. The other group members may deal with her, putting forward the opposing viewpoint. If this does not happen, then the leader needs to intervene, especially if erroneous information is being propounded. Similar tactics to those used when dealing with talkative members can be employed.

The joker
The one who does not take anything seriously. Humour can be useful, but if the subject under discussion is continually trivialized this does detract from the value of the session.

Planning

Neither 'putting her down' nor ignoring her is useful. Acknowledging and, if possible, using something she has said to continue the discussion, or asking her for a further contribution, can help to acknowledge her worth and draw her in.

Most people do not like to stand out in a group. We feel more comfortable if we are 'one of the crowd'. Medical professionals attending antenatal classes may not wish to be singled out, preferring to be considered as an ordinary member of the group.

(f) CONCLUDING

A discussion may naturally draw to a close, but some sort of summary or concluding remarks are helpful. An abrupt stop, 'leaving things in the air', can be rather uncomfortable. If the discussion has been acrimonious, an acknowledgement of the differences of opinion and their validity is helpful in dissipating any negative feelings. Inviting a concluding remark from each member is one possibility, such as 'What I liked/disliked about this session was . . .', 'What I feel I have learned today is . . .', 'What I would like to talk about next time is . . .' One danger of summarizing in too final a way is that you may stop them thinking further about the subject. A discussion which leaves them with food for thought is likely to be more useful.

This is a simplified view of group dynamics, which can be a highly complex interaction of processes and relationships.[37,38,39] Recognize that group members are continually reacting with one another and may take different roles at different times, and that both positive and negative behaviour can be used in a learning situation.

5 Teaching Aids

What is a teaching aid? It can be as sophisticated as a video or as simple as a picture. It can be an object such as a pelvis or it

Planning

can be a baby. It is anything that helps you to convey information to your clients. The best teaching aids are those which convey the information you wish conveyed. This may mean aids that you have made, designed or, at the very least, chosen (see Appendix 1). Your favourite aids may become well used, but presenting aids that are dirty, torn or broken will detract from their value.

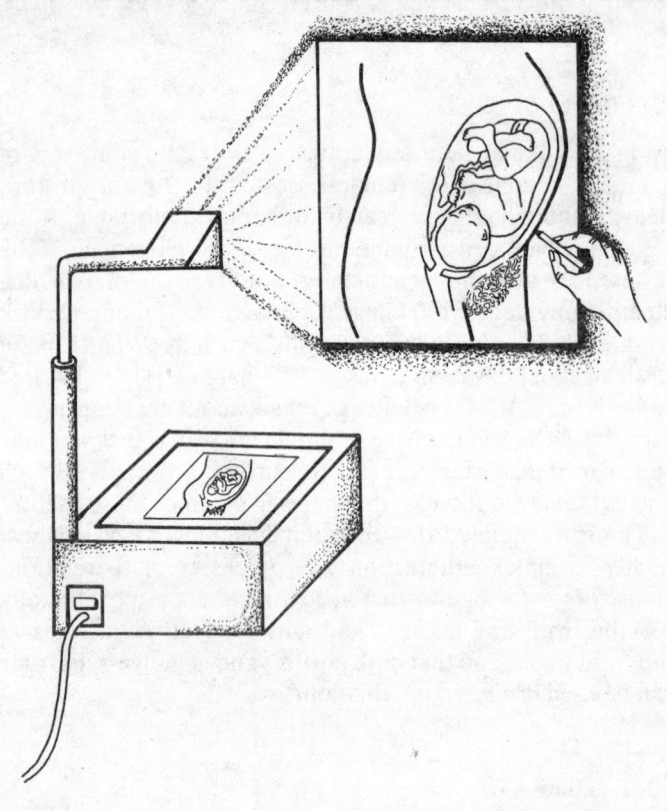

Fig. 3.1 Enlarging a drawing using an overhead projector

Planning

(a) PICTURES

Photographs, book or magazine illustrations, specifically designed flip charts – for example, a birth atlas – may all be useful. If you do not have a suitable picture, a simple drawing may suffice. If you are not a skilled artist, there are some aids which will enable you to convert available resources to your purpose. Often an appropriate picture is too small for class use. It is possible to enlarge using photocopier, overhead projector or pantograph:

Overhead projector
Transfer the drawing you wish to enlarge to a transparency, either by tracing or by a thermal copier, if you have access to a graphics department. Secure a clean sheet of paper to a wall. Project the image on the transparency on to your paper, adjusting the size as desired. Draw round the projected image.

Pantograph
Sometimes called a sketch-a-graph. A simple, cheap but

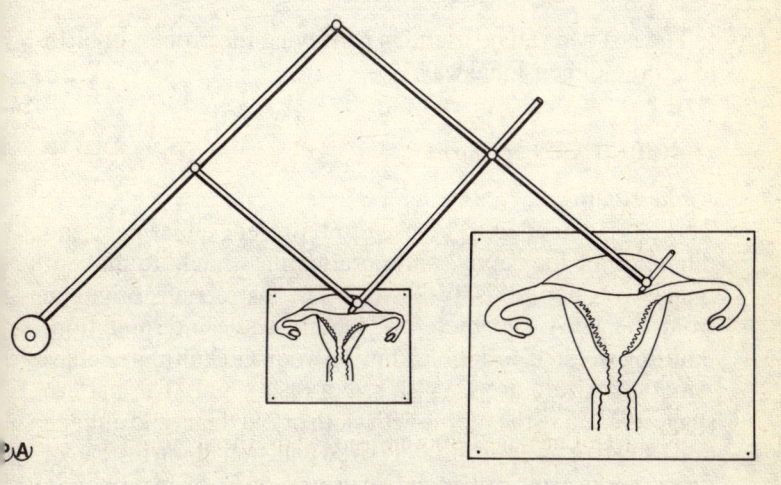

Fig. 3.2 Enlarging a drawing using a pantograph

Planning

effective version can be found in toy shops. More sophisticated models are sold in drawing office supplies shops. It can be used to enlarge, reduce or reproduce a drawing the same size. You will need a piece of hardboard or plywood and drawing pins, paper and pencil. Chalkboard or flip charts can be useful for drawing or noting points during a discussion.

(b) MODELS OR OBJECTS FOR DEMONSTRATION

Layette and other baby equipment.
Feeding bottles and sterilizer.
Pelvis and fetal doll.
Epidural catheter.
Fetal scalp electrode.
Trancutaneous electrical nerve stimulation unit.
Baby doll.
Mother and baby.
Knitted uterus.
Model of pelvic floor.

The last two can be useful in conveying the process of birth in a three-dimensional way.

TEACHING AIDS TO MAKE

Knitted uterus
This aid is intended to be used to represent effacement and dilatation of the cervix, and no attempt is made to make it realistic. A pattern is available.[40] The instructions originate from the USA and therefore require some interpretation: 'knitting worsted' is double knitting wool and knitting needles American size 6 are English size 7 or 4.5 mm. The pattern suggests stuffing the uterus with cloth or old tights and either a doll's head or an appropriately sized ball. A balloon instead of tights works well. You may feel using a doll's head without a

Planning

body looks rather unpleasant and a ball may be more acceptable. A complete doll does not give the correct shape.

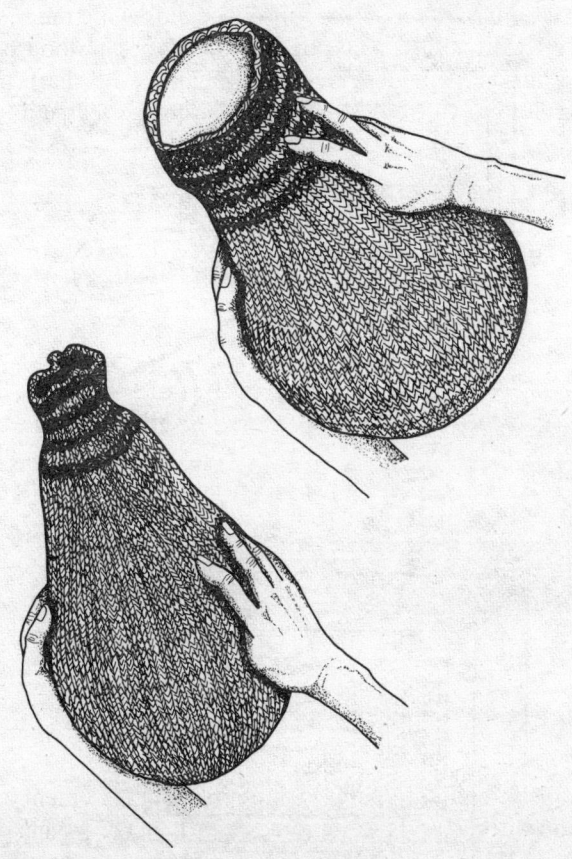

Fig. 3.3 Knitted uterus

Model of pelvic floor
A simulated pelvic floor can be useful for demonstrating the delivery of a baby and the site for episiotomy.[41] This can be made from a plastic bowl or a shoe box. In either, the bottom is removed and replaced with polyurethane foam appropriately

Planning

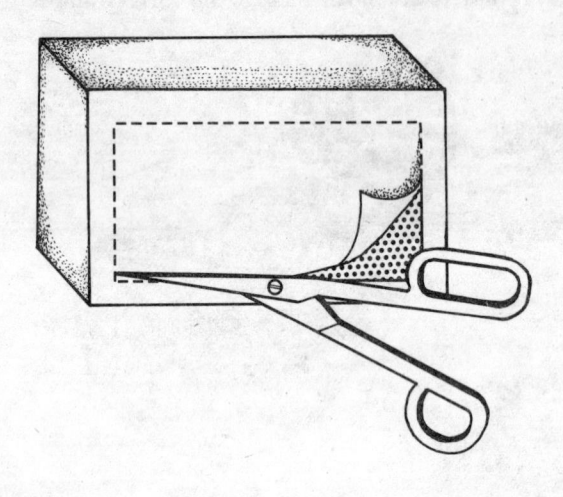

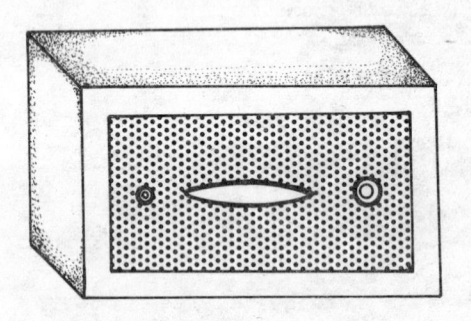

Fig. 3.4 Making a 'shoe-box' pelvic floor

marked and cut. A shoe box is easier to cut, though less realistic. Too much realism, however, may not be desirable. The sight of a doll's head squeezing through an unrealistic, shoe-box pelvic floor can still cause some clients to wince!

Planning

To make the model:

Remove bottom of shoe box, leaving a border an inch wide all round. Cut a piece of one-inch-thick polyurethane foam the same size as the bottom of the box.
Glue foam in place with a universal adhesive (non-oil based).
Mark position of urethra, vagina and anus with a permanent felt-tip marker.
Slit open vaginal opening with craft knife.
If using a plastic bowl, ensure that the base is large enough to allow you to cut a hole for the doll to pass through.
Remove the base with a sharp craft knife.
Cut a circle of foam one inch larger than the hole.
Glue foam in place with a quick-setting epoxy resin.

It can be useful to have two versions of a pelvic floor, one in which the size of the vaginal opening is normal, non-stretched. This can be used to demonstrate what happens when the baby's head first descends on to the perineum. A second version in which the vaginal opening is large enough to permit the passage of a doll can be used to demonstrate delivery.

(c) TECHNICAL AIDS

Overhead projector
This has an advantage over a flip chart or chalk board in that you can maintain eye contact with clients for more of the time. When using the projector, try to ensure that both screen and projector are correctly aligned to avoid the distortion called 'the keystone effect'. This can be avoided if the screen is tilted forward from the top so that it is a few degrees off the vertical. Check that all the clients can see the screen; ensure the projector or your person is not obstructing their view. The noise from a projector fan can interfere with communication, so turn it off when not in use. Transparencies can be prepared in advance, but can also be used to write on during the session.

Planning

The most effective transparencies are simple, brief, use few words, are written in lower-case letters and display no more than three concepts per transparency. Use only the correct pens, of which there are two types: water-based, which can be removed with a damp tissue, and spirit-based, sometimes called 'permanent'. This can be removed with methylated spirit.

Slides
These can be commercially prepared, or made by the teacher; with recorded audio commentary or narration by the teacher.

Films
There are a number of suitable 16 mm films. Some are trigger films, short films of just a few minutes' duration designed to act as a stimulus to discussion.

Video
This is gradually replacing film. Many videos are available, some specifically prepared for health education use. Some television programmes will provide useful material.

If you are using sophisticated equipment, make sure you know how to use it and how to 'trouble-shoot'. Such equipment is also expensive, so it is wise to know what you must not do with it.

If you practise using your aid, whether it is simple or complicated, you will be more confident. If you are narrating slides, practise, not necessarily with a precise script, but by mapping out a plan of what you wish to say. This will help you to avoid hesitation and repetition. Listening to a tape of your narrative can help you to refine and pace your delivery. If you are using a film or video, view it, more than once if possible, and plan what points you can bring out to start a discussion. After you have used it, make a note of the points that interested or confused or upset your clients.

Before every session it is sensible to check your teaching

Planning

aids. Is everything where it is supposed to be, or has someone borrowed it? Aids on loan may have to be ordered well in advance. Is the equipment in working order? Have you spare fuses, bulbs? Has your venue the necessary equipment or facilities? If it proves impossible to use the aid, have you made contingency plans?

(d) LEAFLETS AND POSTERS

Look at them, read them. Do they say what you want them to say? Will the clients understand them? It is possible that slogans on posters are so clever and subtle that the client misses the point. Are the visual images appropriate to the social class and culture of your client group? If not the message will not be received. Look at the amount of writing on a poster. Consider the length of time a client may look at it; an average time is likely to be fifteen seconds.

There are a number of tests which may be applied to the written material in health education literature to determine the readability. One such formula is the Gobbledegook Test.[42] Most of these tests work on the basis that prose with a long average sentence length and containing many words with three or more syllables will not be understood by the majority of the public. These formulae are only a rough guide and it is advisable to test the material you propose to use on a sample of your clients.

6 Working With Other People

Last but not least, you may be working with other professionals. You may be part of a system where other professionals already take a regular part; such as an obstetric physiotherapist, health visitor, dietitian, obstetrician, paediatrician. If they are not involved, can you suggest they contribute? A team approach will bring a wider range of skills and

Planning

experience to benefit the clients.[43,44,45,46] Think who else might be able to make a contribution to your classes. A National Childbirth Trust breastfeeding counsellor, a Road-Safety Officer or anyone else?

7 Lesson Plans

It is helpful to have a written plan of your work. Start with your aims and objectives, and from these decide the content of the session. Plan appropriate methods and strategies. Note any teaching aids you will require. Timing a session can be difficult, especially when you seek client participation. It is useful if your plan includes some time allocation for different parts of the session, but with flexibility built in. It may be useful to note where you would like to be at the halfway point in the session. If you then find you are running behind your schedule, you can decide what essential items you wish to cover and what may be left out. A lesson plan should also include checks on learning you will use during the session to assist in assessment and evaluation. These activities will effect future planning (see Chapter 1).

A lesson plan written in the form of a grid can help you to take an overall view of the form of your session. For example:

Subject: Buying baby equipment and safety in the home.
Time available: One hour.
Aim: Mothers will be able to make safe preparations for the baby.
Objectives: Mothers will be able to:
  Recall the safety factors to be taken into account when buying baby clothes and equipment.
  Identify possible hazards in the home.
  Demonstrate willingness to make any adaptations needed in the home.
  List considerations of her own health and comfort she should remember when buying equipment.

Planning

Table 3.1 A lesson plan in the form of a grid

Time	Content	Methods and strategies	Checks on learning	Teaching aids
3 mins	Introduce subject	Lecture and discussion	Ask questions throughout	
12 mins	Essential baby equipment	Discussion		Layette pictures of equipment
12 mins	Choosing safely	Lecture and discussion		Safety leaflets
12 mins	Hazards in the home	Demonstration discussion		Video
12 mins	Preventing back strain by careful buying and use of equipment	Demonstration discussion		
5 mins	Summary	Ask questions	Quiz	Worksheet for quiz

TEACHING NOTES

Teaching notes are helpful, especially for the inexperienced teacher. They are an aid to memory, not a script, so keep them brief. Key words, either in capitals, in a different colour or underlined, will help you to quickly find your place.

8 Checklist for Planning

What are your aims and objectives?
Have you all necessary information for the subject?

Planning

Who are your clients and what are their particular needs?
How long will your session last?
Have you planned your methods and strategies?
What aids will you need?
Have your written your teaching notes?
Where will you teach and what are the facilities?
Are your plans flexible?
What needs to be changed next time?

References

1. Maloney, R. (1985), 'Childbirth education classes: expectant parents' expectations,' *Journal of Obstetric, Gynaecological and Neonatal Nurses*, vol. 14, no. 3, May/June, pp. 245–8.
2. Draper, J., Field, S., Kerr, M. and Hare, M. J. (1982), 'The level of preparedness for parenthood', *Maternal and Child Health*, February, pp. 44–7.
3. Taylor, A. (1985), 'Antenatal classes and the consumer: mothers' and fathers' views', *Health Education Journal*, vol. 44, no. 2, pp 79–82.
4. Thompson, H. (1982), 'Antenatal care: what about father?' *Nursing Times. Community Outlook*, vol. 78, no. 15, 14 April, pp. 99–104.
5. Draper *et al.* 'The level of preparedness for parenthood'.
6. Adams, L. (1982), 'Consumers' views of antenatal education', *Health Education Journal*, vol. 41, no. 1, pp. 12–16.
7. Gould, D. (1986), 'Locally organised antenatal classes and their effectiveness', *Nursing Times*, vol. 82, no. 45, 5 November, pp. 59–61.
8. Webber, A. and Janzen R. (1982), 'Antenatal education – Does it work?', *Midwives Chronicle*, vol. 95, no. 1130, March, pp. 94–7.
9. Taylor, 'Antenatal classes and the consumer'.
10. Draper *et al.*, 'The level of preparedness for parenthood'.
11. Gould, 'Locally organised antenatal classes and their effectiveness'.
12. Adams, 'Consumers' views of antenatal education'.
13. Webber and Janzen, 'Antenatal education – Does it work?'
14. Taylor, 'Antenatal classes and the consumer'.
15. Adams, 'Consumers' views of antenatal education'.
16. Gould, 'Locally organized antenatal classes and their effectiveness'.
17. Taylor, 'Antenatal classes and the consumer'.
18. Adams, 'Consumers' views of antenatal education'.
19. Gould, 'Locally organized antenatal classes and their effectiveness'.
20. Webber and Janzen, 'Antenatal education – Does it work?'

Planning

21 McIntosh, J. (1988), 'A consumer view of birth preparation classes: attitudes of a sample of working-class primiparae', *Midwives Chronicle*, vol. 101, no. 1200, January, pp. 8–9.

22 WHO, (1985), 'Health promotion. A discussion document on the concept and principles', *International Journal of Health Education*, vol. 23, no. 1.

23 Postman, N. and Weingartner, C. (1969), *Teaching as a Subversive Activity*, Penguin, Harmondsworth, pp. 28–35.

24 Antenatal Language Kit. To teach English for pregnancy, Commission for Racial Equality (see Appendix 1).

25 Relaxation Classes for Pregnant Women. Booklet of sign language, Rycote Centre for the Deaf (see Appendix 1).

26 Evans, G. and Parker, P. (1985), 'Preparing teenagers for parenthood', *Midwives Chronicle*, vol. 98, no. 1172, September, pp. 239–40.

27 Todd, J. E., Lapthorn, J. and McIntosh, J. (1988), 'Teenage Club at the Royal Berkshire', *Midwives Chronicle*, vol. 101, no. 1207, August, pp. 238–41.

28 Watson, G. (1988), 'Parentcraft for single girls', *Midwives Chronicle*, vol. 101, no. 1210, November, pp. 346–7.

29 Grayshon, J. (1989), 'Special delivery?' *Midwives Chronicle*, vol. 102, no. 1212, January, pp. 12–13.

30 Fraser, J. (1987), 'Parenthood education for adoptive parents', *Midwives Chronicle*, vol. 100, no. 1196, September, pp. 276–8.

31 Jaques, D. (1984), *Learning in Groups*, Croom Helm, London, p. xi.

32 *Ibid.* pp. 116–22.

33 Simkin, P. (1988), 'Role play of labor: a unique and valuable childbirth education technique', *International Journal of Childbirth Education*, vol. 3, no. 2, pp. 14–15.

34 Jacques, D. (1984), *Learning in Groups*, Croom Helm, London, pp. 136–8.

35 *Ibid.*, pp. 140–2.

36 Brown, A. (1986), *Groupwork*, 2nd edn, Gower, Aldershot, pp. 52–8.

37 Jacques, *Learning in Groups*, pp. 1–61.

38 Brown, *Groupwork*, pp. 70–6.

39 Kitzinger, S. (1977), *Education and Counselling for Childbirth*, Baillière Tindall, London, pp. 32–53.

40 Knitted Uterus Pattern available from: ACPOG, Mrs A. Hallatt, 33 Twyford Close, Cramlington, Northumberland, NE23 9PH (20p + 19p p&p).

41 Kitzinger, *Education and Counselling for Childbirth*, p. 69.

42 Ewles, L. and Simnett, I. (1985), *Promoting Health. A Practical Guide to Health Education*, Wiley, Chichester, pp. 190–1.

43 The Association of Chartered Physiotherapists in Obstetrics and

Planning

Gynaecology (1987), 'Working together in psychophysical preparation for childbirth', *ACPOG Journal*, no. 61, July, p. 4.
44 Black, T., Booth, K. and Faulkner, A. (1984), 'Co-operation or conflict?', *Senior Nurse*, 14 November, vol. 1, no. 33, pp. 25–6.
45 Fraser, J. (1988), 'Parenthood education – where are we now?', *Midwives Chronicle*, vol. 101, no. 1210, November, pp. 345–7.
46 Hammond, N., Dyas, G. and Plaut, J. (1986), 'Doing away with "us and them" parentcraft classes', *Midwives Chronicle*, vol. 99, no. 1177, February, pp. 42–3.

Further Reading

Abercrombie, M. L. J. and Terry, P. M. (1978), *Talking to Learn. Improving Teaching and Learning in Small Groups*, Society for Research into Higher Education, University of Surrey, Guildford, Surrey.

Delafleur, T. P. and Payne, J. D. (1981), 'Role playing in childbirth education classes', *Maternal and Child Nursing*, vol. 6, September/October, pp. 333–6.

Douglas, T. (1978), *Basic Groupwork*, Tavistock, London.

Fast, J. (1971), *Body Language*, Pan, London.

Hyde, B. I. (1981), 'Curriculum planning for antenatal education', *Nurse Education Today*, vol. 1, no. 6, December, pp. 8–10.

Jacoby, A. (1988), 'Mothers' views about information and advice in pregnancy and childbirth: findings from a national study', *Midwifery*, vol. 4, pp. 103–10.

McCann, R. (1985), *Graphics Handbook: An Introduction to Design and Printing for the Non-specialist*, Health Education Council, National Extension College.

Munro, J. (1988), 'Parentcraft classes with Bengali mothers', *Health Visitor*, vol. 61, no. 2, February, p. 48.

Perkins, E. R. (1980), *Education for Childbirth and Parenthood*, Croom Helm, London.

Powell, L. S. (1978), *A Guide to the Use of Visual Aids*, BACIE, 16 Park Crescent, London WIN 4AP.

Van Ments, M. (1983), *The Effective Use of Role-Play. A Handbook for Teachers and Trainers*, Kogan Page, London.

Williams, M. and Booth, D. (1985), *Antenatal Education. Guidelines for Teachers*, 3rd edn, Churchill Livingstone, Edinburgh.

4
Partners

When you formulate your aims and objectives for teaching partners you need to ask yourself whether you are looking at it from the standpoint of the partner's own needs or the woman's needs. If you think of the couple as a unit, consider at times there may be conflicting needs within that unit. Partners are sometimes thought of only as labour coaches. If you take a wider approach to their possible role in pregnancy, birth and afterwards, this can help to enhance the couple's experience of this period in their lives and their future relationship.

In this chapter the 'partner' is taken to be the woman's male consort. It is well to bear in mind, however, that she may be supported through her pregnancy, labour and after the birth by her parents, other relative or female friend. Whoever is chosen by the mother deserves the opportunity to learn in an appropriate manner.

1 What Are Your Aims?

That he will be able to:

Show a supportive attitude during pregnancy.
Give practical and emotional support to his partner during labour.
Cope adequately with the experience of labour.
Be prepared for a changing role.
Understand the help he can give the mother after birth.

Partners

Enjoy the birth of their child.
Or . . .

Having your aims in mind,

2 What are Your Objectives?

At the end of the session/course he will be able to:

List his partner's health needs in pregnancy.
Demonstrate recognition of his partner's emotional needs in pregnancy.
Recall the process of labour.
Recall the coping strategies his partner can use in labour.
Demonstrate recognition of the role he can play in labour support.
Demonstrate confidence in his ability to be of help to his partner.
Discuss his own hopes and fears about labour.
Discuss the changes a baby may bring to a relationship.
Demonstrate the ability to change a nappy.
Or . . .

3 What Are You Going To Teach?

What do partners want from classes? Research has shown they want information; hard facts on birth and babies. They also want positive guidance about helping in labour, and those that do attend are more likely to feel afterwards they have been useful.[1,2,3] Assistance in labour is not their only role. Their support in pregnancy can positively influence a mother's health and peace of mind. Partners may not always wish to attend classes. In retrospect they may regret not having had more knowledge about birth and on emotional needs and

Partners

adjustment of priorities after the birth. But they may not see the need for such information antenatally. Your advertising and invitations should make it clear that they are both welcomed and that their needs are taken into account. What men do not want is condescension, to be thought of as unintelligent and to be treated as 'humpers of furniture and butts of staff jokes'.[4]

(a) PREGNANCY

Think how the men may feel about pregnancy. They may be elated at the thought of a much wanted baby; or they may be thinking, 'I want this baby but how will we manage the mortgage?' Or, 'We shall have to move and the council said no flat for two years; why did she have to get pregnant!'. Or, 'I'm too young to be a father, I want to go out and have fun'. The assumption that all is happiness and joy may leave them feeling resentful and a simple statement from you recognizing that feelings about the pregnancy may be mixed can help. You have acknowledged the validity of their feelings and this can free them to think about their partner.

Consider what men need to know about pregnancy. It can be helpful for them to understand the effect the growing fetus will have on her whole body (see Chapter 4). The phenomenon of morning sickness is well known, but not so well known is that it can be evening sickness, or even all-day sickness. The physical changes of early pregnancy are not always obvious. He may not be prepared for the tiredness in early pregnancy that leaves her too exhausted to go out with him in the evening. He will probably help with the shopping and heavy lifting jobs when she is large and cumbersome, but will not realize that the effects of loosened ligaments means that she may need help before she even looks pregnant, or that the fact that she has dropped half the plates they possessed could be caused by carpal tunnel syndrome. You cannot expect him to be able to recite a list of all the minor problems

Partners

of pregnancy. If, however, he can be aware of the multiplicity of changes which may occur he can be better prepared to cope with them.

How does the woman's partner feel now she is pregnant? She is the one who has 'the burden and privilege of pregnancy'.[5] He cannot take part in it; her physical and emotional needs are the focus of attention, she is the one who looks pregnant, but he is becoming a parent too. He has to make emotional adjustments and changes in his life. Pregnant women gain support from each other, but because he is not obviously pregnant there may be less opportunity for him to share his feelings with other pregnant fathers. You may not be able to arrange a discussion, but it may be some comfort for him to know that others share his feelings and he may be more able to broach the subject with friends. How does he feel physically? It is possible for men to display physical symptoms during pregnancy and labour, and while it probably is not necessary to describe the more bizarre forms of the couvade syndrome, it may relieve his mind to know that it is not uncommon.

It can be difficult for the partner to cope with her emotional changes. Maybe his normally efficient, totally in control wife becomes absent minded. If she is on a 'high' one day, weeping the next, and biting his head off the day after that, it probably is part of the normal labile emotions of pregnancy. He may find it hard to take, but at least he knows the possible reason. When she looks and feels like a beached whale at the end of pregnancy, how may she feel and how may he feel about the way she looks? Is she blooming, feeling very special and good about herself? Or hating every minute of being pregnant, feeling grotesque and wishing it was all over. He may think her pregnant body is very beautiful or is looking forward to her regaining her figure. Humour can help, but with sensitivity. One too many jokes about 'the elephant I married' may send her into floods of tears.

A pregnant woman will benefit from her partner's support

Partners

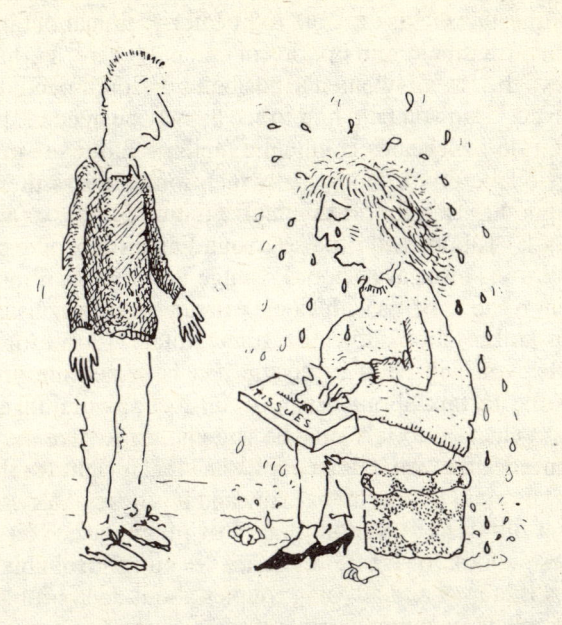

'I trod on an ant! It's dead!'

in maintaining or improving her health. If he understands that smoking is detrimental, perhaps they could give up together. If he knows what alcohol can do to babies he will not chide her for being unsociable when she refuses to drink lager in the pub. He may not be able, through financial constraints, to make many changes in their lifestyle but knowledge can enable him to maximize their resources. Fathers may request advice on equipment and preparation at home. Perhaps you can reassure him that you will not be advising her to buy up the complete contents of the baby shop (see Chapter 5). He can be important as a mediator and advocate for her if she finds

Partners

doctors and hospitals intimidating. You can help him to know what questions to ask to obtain the information about investigations, treatment and options in antenatal care. Perhaps he thinks 'this is all women's business, I don't need to get involved.' Can you help him to see he may be needed?

Men do experience conflicting feelings about sex in pregnancy.[6] Doctors do not usually mention it unless there is a very good reason for abstaining from intercourse, so who do men ask? Taboos and rituals surrounding birth form a part of all cultures.[7] But as societies change and formal rituals disappear it can leave us with vague worries about what is 'right'. Sex is still a taboo subject in some situations and for some people; you will need to decide if it is something you are prepared to talk about. Even if you feel shy or judge your clients reluctant to talk, maybe you could just give them the reassurance that what as a couple they feel is right for them is OK. They will not harm the baby and it is normal for couples to feel different at various stages of pregnancy. You could suggest a book for future reference.[8] You are probably not a sexual therapist and advising couples about deep problems is not within your competence, but some general comments and advice could be given. Perhaps the most important fact is for them to be prepared for changes. Some physical changes may not be obvious; her breast tenderness may preclude caressing during lovemaking and there will almost certainly be changes in libido in both partners.[9] Her desire may increase or decrease at different times during pregnancy, and she may possibly feel very 'unsexy' and unattractive when she is large. His feelings can also increase or decrease as pregnancy advances, the mother image seeming incompatible with the lover image to some men at this time. If the increased desire in one partner is not reciprocated this obviously can be a problem. Can you encourage them to talk about their feelings? Communication is always important in a relationship and especially at a time of change. Encourage them to tell each other what they like or dislike, to say, 'just because I don't want intercourse doesn't mean I don't love you'. Humour can be a help too and some couples would say it was essential when considering sex, especially in later pregnancy. Men may have fears for themselves, fearing damage to the penis by the baby. However bizarre, these fears are nonetheless real. Men also have fears for their babies, fears of harming baby or starting premature labour. Although this is unlikely,[10] if a premature labour is a probability, advice to abstain avoids guilt feelings should this occur. Sexual activity may well decline in the last few weeks through tiredness and general discomfort. Sex, of course does not have to mean full intercourse and this can be a positive factor in their relationship.[11] You do not have to be explicit if you mention this. Couples can use their imaginations if you suggest they can discover new ways of enjoying one another. There are many books available on sexual techniques should they feel the need of new ideas. Semen contains prostaglandins,[12] which are also used medically to ripen the cervix at the end of pregnancy. Intercourse, with nipple stimulation, may be a pleasant way of encouraging labour to start when the estimated date of delivery has passed.

Relaxation is taught to mothers antenatally but fathers should also be taught. Learning the technique will enable him to support her and he can gain benefit for himself. Pregnant or not we all have stresses in our lives and the ability to relax can mitigate the effects of that stress (see Chapter 6). Touch can play a part when teaching relaxation to couples. They can be helped to discover tension in each other, and ways in which they can work together to release it.[13,14] Touch is a natural and instinctive way of comforting and calming, but sensitivity to individual reactions is essential.[15] Touching one another in public may not be acceptable.

(b) LABOUR AND BIRTH

The general trend is for the mother to have a labour companion of her choice. This may or may not be the father of the

Partners

child. Does every couple want to be together at this time? Couples should not be given the impression that they are unusual or in some way wrong if they do not wish it. Some women may prefer a female companion; this is the norm in many cultures. Think about why partners attend the birth. Is it to coach or assist the mother to cope with labour or to witness and share the birth of their child? One father said, 'I was there at conception, during pregnancy and the first part of labour. I felt if I had left then it would have been like walking out after three acts of a four-act play, then reading the reviews later!' Many fathers find attending the birth of their child a wonderful and fulfilling experience. However, fathers who attend the birth without preparation may not be so happy.[16] Indeed every labour companion should have the chance to become familiar with the coping strategies taught to the mother and the venue, procedures and options the mother will encounter. Consider whether you should attempt to persuade fathers to attend. They may show reluctance because they have very understandable worries about how they will cope in an unknown situation and alien environment. Fears of fainting, of looking foolish and unmanly, of seeing her in pain and being unable to do anything to help; all these feelings may make them feel it would be better to let the experts get on with the job. If we can show them how they can help and how important their presence can be, maybe they will overcome their reluctance and become a willing labour companion. If, however, gentle encouragement becomes coercion, unnecessary anxieties may result. While the birth is an important event in a father's as well as mother's life, it is a small part of life. Helping men to make the transition to fatherhood may be more important than their presence in the delivery room.

Labour can be a stressful time for men as well as women. Knowing the practicalities of when, where and how to get to hospital can help to give them confidence when she says 'It's started.' The birth of their baby may be a fantastic experience and they may expect this. Do they also expect, during labour,

Partners

to be bored, scared, embarrassed or tired? They may appreciate some 'self-preservation tips for fathers'. For example, you could offer advice about the clothing to wear in the heat of the labour ward. They may need sustenance during a long labour, knowing whether facilities are available in or near the hospital or if they will need to provide for themselves will be useful.

Teaching the breathing techniques for labour to the father is important because it is easy in the stress of labour for the mother to forget (see Chapter 6). The comfort of his physical presence is often very important to her. It may not come easily to him to cuddle her in public, but given encouragement that it is acceptable and desirable, hopefully, he will overcome his inhibitions. Some women may use vocalization as a way of coping with labour contractions. It is easy, in this circumstance, for attendants to assume a level of distress greater than the woman will acknowledge. It can be helpful if the partner is aware of this. Warn him also that in labour she may change. For example, she may intensely dislike the type of back massage she found so soothing antenatally. Or she may become aggressive or irrational at times. Reassure him that, regardless of her behaviour, she does need his support.

To support her, knowledge of the process of labour and the routine procedures she will undergo will be useful to him (see Chapter 7). If the hospital has restrictions on his presence during any procedure, it will probably be less distressing for them both if they realize this in advance and also the reasons for such restrictions. Should they find those reasons unacceptable and wish to challenge them, discussing this with a senior member of staff in advance, rather than in the heat of the moment, is more likely to result in a satisfactory outcome.

Where will he be at the moment of birth? Arm round her or close by her shoulder, encouraging, touching; or down at the end of the bed shouting encouragement from the touchline, or snapping away with his camera to capture the moment on film? Are cameras allowed in the delivery room?

Partners

It is reasonable to prepare him for the possibility of resuscitation of the baby. He is more likely than the mother to be close to the action when this happens. He may find intubation less disturbing if he has received an explanation beforehand. However, it is as well to bear in mind that he may not be receptive to such information because he has the expectation of a normal birth with no problems. Couples should be encouraged to expect that soon after the birth they will have the opportunity to be alone with their baby and each other for a while.

(c) AFTER BIRTH

Fathers can be very unprepared for the tremendous impact a baby can have upon the life of a couple. They accept there will be changes: that mother will spend time caring for the baby, baby sitters will need to be arranged before they can go out together, and possibly they may have to curtail some hobbies. However, until they have experienced this, it can be difficult to envisage the way a baby completely takes over a household. Life is never going to be the same again. Being prepared can help the couple make adjustments.

If the physical and emotional changes the mother will experience after birth are explained to the partner this can help him provide the support and understanding she needs (see Chapter 9). There is an expectation, when the six-week postnatal check has been carried out and all is pronounced normal, that the mother will be as she was before pregnancy. This of course is not so; a sutured perineum may not yet be comfortable, a Caesarean will not allow vigorous physical activity for some time, abdominal muscles are still slack and ligaments will take up to five months to return to normal. The baby blues may be over but postnatal depression can be a problem. It is important the partner has some knowledge and understanding of postnatal depression so he is able to offer her appropriate help. Depression can cause an individual to close

Partners

in on herself and render her unable to seek the help she needs. His knowledge of who to contact may then be invaluable to her.

Think about how the father may feel after the birth. Happy and proud of his part in the creation of a new life, content in his new role as a father? Or resentful of the baby because his partner seems to have no time for him and his needs, jealous of the close and special relationship between mother and baby, or depressed himself, daunted by the responsibility he has taken on? You can encourage him to share his feelings with his partner, his friends or family. The relationship with his partner will be different, she is now the mother of his child and between them they are responsible for a third person. If he knows the necessary adjustments may take time, he will be more able to cope with conflicting emotions should they occur.

Changing attitudes in society to parenthood/fatherhood can create uncertainties for men.[17] The trend in the western world is for fathers to be actively involved with their children from birth. Styles of parenting vary under influences of culture, family tradition, personal inclination and necessity. Discussions with others may help them begin to discover their own style of parenting. Fathers can, and of course do, play an active role in the development of their children but sometimes need active encouragement in the early days. Men are often frightened of harming small babies by inexpert handling and not keen on demonstrating their own incompetence. Babies' needs can be discussed (see Chapter 8). Practical help can really only be given once the baby has arrived, but antenatally he can be prepared to expect and seek active involvement. The father–child bond can thereby be enhanced.[18]

(d)..

Can you think of anything else a woman's partner may need or want to know?

Partners

4 How Will you Teach

Think about the different ways partners may be included in classes.

A complete course for couples.
One class of the course for couples.
A men-only class.

You may be running daytime classes which working men cannot attend. Try to organize one in the evening for them. One class only will not allow you to build a relationship with them and some subjects may not be feasible, for example discussions on sex. Some subjects may have to be covered less thoroughly than you ideally would wish, but you will be able to give some basic advice and give them the opportunity to ask questions.

Think whether some subjects are best covered with women alone or some with men alone. It may seem ideal to teach them together but women may defer to men in this situation and not feel as free as they might to put forward their own opinions. Consider whether you should invite partners if only some can come. Partnerless (for whatever reason) women may not feel comfortable if they are in a minority. It may be culturally unacceptable for some women to be in the presence of strange men, especially if their own husbands are not present.

Women may feel happier to discuss their problems and to exhibit their ungainliness when exercising if men are not present.

Men-only classes are less common but can allow men to share worries they would be reluctant to speak of if their womenfolk were present. Inhibitions can be less when it is 'all boys together'.

The information men want and need is similar to that for women but the emphasis may be different. Try to find out

Partners

from the men what they want to know. Feelings men experience about pregnancy, childbirth, attending classes and being a father are so variable it would be a foolhardy antenatal teacher who assumed she knew what her clients wanted. Most antenatal teachers are women; how can we really know how men feel? To increase your own understanding you can talk to a father; your own, another relative, your spouse or a friend.[19]

You may be able to invite to the class a couple who have recently became parents to discuss their experiences and feelings.

Demonstration and practice of relaxation and breathing techniques are usual. Some problems can be encountered here if you have a 'joker'. It may be that he is unable to take it seriously or it may be sheer embarrassment. Humour on your part may help to overcome this (see group work, Chapter 3).

If you are expecting couples to touch each other in public you will need to use tact and some skill when initiating this activity. A relationship may not have included this type of activity before, or intimacy of this kind could be embarrassing for them in public.

Role play may be appropriate with some groups. Rehearsing the support for the labouring mother can be a vivid way of learning the skill and a way of working through their own feelings.[20]

A chance to visit the labour ward is usually appreciated by the fathers.

It will be useful to consider many of the factors discussed in this chapter whether the partners are present or not. If you are teaching the women alone, most will have a man in their lives and you can help them to prepare their partners.

Partners

5 What Aids Can You Use?

All the aids noted in other chapters relevant to the subjects discussed.

One aid common to many 'father's evenings' is a film or video of a birth or births. Look at them very carefully before you show one. Think what your aims and objectives are. Do the fathers want to see a film? Could you ask them? Could you show films you propose to use first to a non-medical male friend or family member? Then you can decide if any one really fulfils its purpose.

6 Trigger Questions for Discussion

Would you like to tell me why you have come to antenatal classes?
What do you expect to gain from the antenatal classes?
What physical changes have you noticed in her so far?
What have her emotions been like since she has been pregnant?
Is there anything about her antenatal care that concerns you?
Were you with her when she had her ultrasound scan?
What were your feeling when you saw it?
What do you expect to be doing when she is in labour?
Labour contractions can be painful. How do you think you would feel seeing her in pain?
What do you think you can do to help her in labour?
What have other fathers told you about being present in labour?
Is there anything in particular about labour or the birth that worries you?
Have you seen a birth on television?
What was the nicest thing about it?
What was the worst thing about it?

Partners

What changes do you think a baby is going to make to your life?
What are you looking forward to doing for your baby?

7 How will you know when you have achieved your aims and objectives?

Discussion in class can give you some feedback.
Questionnaires may have a role.
Can you arrange a reunion at a time when fathers can attend?

Suggested Leaflets

Seel, R. (1984), *Becoming a Father*, National Childbirth Trust, London. (1986), *A Guide to Labour for Expectant Parents*, National Childbirth Trust, London.

References

1 Taylor, A. (1985), 'Antenatal classes and the consumer: mothers' and fathers' views', *Health Education Journal*, vol. 44, no. 2, pp. 79–82.
2 Maloney, R. (1985), 'Childbirth education classes: expectant parents' expectations', *Journal of Obstetric, Gynaecological and Neonatal Nurses*, vol. 14, no. 3, May/June, pp. 245–8.
3 Thompson, H. (1982), 'Antenatal care. What about Father?' *Nursing Times. Community Outlook*, vol. 78, no. 15, 14 April, pp. 99–104.
4 Taylor, 'Antenatal classes and the consumer'.
5 Francis, M. (1986), *Fathering for Men. Every Man's Guide to the First Years of Parenthood*, Generation, Bristol, p. 9.
6 Seel, R. (1987), *The Uncertain Father*, Gateway, Bath, pp. 43–6.
7 Kitzinger, S. (1977), *Education and Counselling for Childbirth*, Baillière Tindall, London, pp. 205–6.
8 Bing, E. and Colman, L. (1978), *Making Love During Pregnancy*, Bantam, London.
9 Falicov, C. J. (1973) 'Sexual adjustment during first pregnancy and post partum', *American Journal of Obstetrics and Gynecology*, vol. 117, no. 7, 1 December, pp. 991–1000.
10 Perkins, R. P. (1979), 'Sexual behaviour and response in relation to applications of pregnancy', *American Journal of Obstetrics and Gynecology*, vol. 134, no. 5, July, pp. 498–505.

Partners

11 Roeber, J. (1987), *Shared Parenthood*, Century, London, pp. 42–4.
12 Speroff, L. and Ramwell, P. W. (1970), 'Prostaglandins in reproductive physiology', *American Journal of Obstetrics and Gynecology*, vol. 107, 1 August, pp. 1111–30.
13 Madders, J. (1979), *Stress and Relaxation*, Macdonald Optima, London, pp. 28–31.
14 Dale, B. and Roeber, J. (1982), *Exercises for Childbirth*, Century, London, pp. 78–87.
15 Kitzinger, S. (1987), *Education and Counselling for Childbirth*, London, pp. 156–64.
16 Thompson, 'Antenatal care. What about Father?'
17 Seel, R. (1987), *The Uncertain Father*, pp. 1–12.
18 Hutchins, P. and Harvey, D. (1977), 'A supplement on parentcraft. The father's role', *Nursing Mirror*, vol. 145, no. 13, 29 September, pp. v–xii.
19 Pearson, J. and O'Brien, M. (1987), 'Reach out and touch the fathers in your classes', *New Generation*, vol. 6, no. 2, June, pp. 19–20.
20 Simkin, P. (1988), 'Role play of labor: a unique and valuable childbirth education technique', *International Journal of Childbirth Education*, vol. 3, no. 2, pp. 14–15.

Further Reading

Bailey, V. R. (1989), 'Sexuality – before and after birth', *Midwives Chronicle*, vol. 102, no. 1212, January, pp. 24–6.
Balaskas, J. (1984), *The Active Birth Partner's Handbook*, Sidgwick and Jackson, London.
Bozett, F. and Hanson, S. (1986), 'Focus on fathers', *Nursing Times*, vol. 82, no. 11, 12 March, pp. 38–40.
Cobb, J. (1980), *Babyshock*, Arrow, London.
Kitzinger, S. (1987), *Freedom and Choice in Childbirth*, Viking Penguin, Harmondsworth, pp. 96–7.
Lewis, C. (1986), *Becoming a Father*, Open University, Milton Keynes.
Lewis, C. (1987), *Reassessing Fatherhood*, Sage, London.
Mueller, L. S. (1985), 'Pregnancy and Sexuality', *Journal of Obstetric, Gynaecological and Neonatal Nurses*, vol. 14, no. 4, pp. 289–94.
Ritchie, J. E. (1970), 'The father's role in family-centred childbirth', *Midwife and Health Visitor*, vol. 6, August, pp. 302–7.

5
Pregnancy

This chapter covers a variety of subjects which may be taught at different sessions, but for convenience are considered together. You need to think about the timing of the items. For example, when will you teach about nutrition, alcohol and smoking? Teaching these early in pregnancy will assist clients to gain maximum benefit from the learning. An antenatal teacher can not hope to think of every question mothers may wish to ask about pregnancy. If you can create an accepting ambience and allow enough time for discussion, hopefully mothers will feel able to voice their worries and queries.

1 What Are Your Aims?

Clients will be able to:

Show understanding of the purposes of antenatal care.
Make the necessary changes to ensure a healthy lifestyle.
Recall their rights in relation to work and benefits.
Show knowledge of the minor disorders of pregnancy.
Make informed judgements about buying baby equipment and safety in the home.
Or . . . ?

Having your aims in mind,

Pregnancy

2 What Are Your Objectives?

At the end of the session the mother will be able to:

Demonstrate a willingness to improve her diet.
Recall the steps she has to take to obtain her due benefits.
Identify symptoms of potential problems which should be reported to a doctor.
Demonstrate exercises to improve suppleness.
Demonstrate exercises to relieve backache.
Demonstrate correct lifting techniques.
Recall the effects of alcohol and tobacco smoking on the fetus.
List the factors with which to judge the safety of baby equipment.
Or . . . ?

3 What Will You Teach?

(a) FETAL DEVELOPMENT

Consider what information clients may want and what would be useful for them to know about the way a fetus develops and grows: how big or heavy it is at different stages of pregnancy or what it does or what it is capable of sensing. A discussion of fetal movements usually occurs and this can be a suitable time to introduce the idea of movements as an indicator of fetal well-being. Those not aware of movements until later than average may need reassurance. It can also be helpful for them to realize that the fetus will have periods of rest and activity. Think about the advice you could give on what to do if movements are absent or considerably reduced. Multiparae or those in later pregnancy may offer their own experiences of fetal reactions to noise, including music.[1] Being able to visualize what their baby looks like at different stages of gestation can help mothers to identify with the growing fetus, giving pleasure and helping them to adjust to the changes pregnancy brings.

Mothers are concerned about possible harm to the fetus. It is useful to discuss the role of the placenta in nourishing and protecting the fetus. You could introduce the idea of the placenta as a sieve rather than a complete barrier, alerting them to possible dangers they can avoid. It may be appropriate to talk of what can be done to help babies who are born with problems or born before they are due.

(b) NUTRITION

A dietitian may be available to teach this but if not, you need to think about what aspects you can discuss. Before talking of any changes in the diet necessary for pregnancy, a review of a balanced or healthy diet can be a useful starting point. This is after all, an opportunity for long-term health improvement not to be missed. The particular nutritional needs of pregnancy, such as iron and folate and calcium requirements can be covered.[2] You may need to dispel the 'eating for two' myth. Many will be anxious not to gain too much weight and will be encouraged to take care in pregnancy because of the difficulty some women experience in losing excessive weight after the birth. However, because we live in a society which equates slimness with beauty, advice may need to be given to women who are either underweight or may eat a diet in pregnancy below the optimum for good fetal growth, doing this in an attempt to preserve their appearance. Average or appropriate weight gains for pregnancy are quoted by many authorities such as obstetricians and nutritionists, but this is not necessarily useful knowledge for pregnant women. It is better that they have a good understanding of different food groups and how to construct a healthy diet rather than worrying about what the scales will read next time they visit the clinic.

Pregnancy

Discussing the theoretical ideal diet may not be helpful if individual differences in taste, custom, income and cooking facilities are ignored. Vegetarians and vegans have societies able to advise on nutrition in pregnancy (see Appendix 1). Different cultural or religious groups,[3] those on low incomes or living in 'bed sits' or bed and breakfast accommodation, have different needs. It can be beneficial for the whole group to share in this more specific information. Since vegetarian sources of protein are cheaper than meat, those on a low budget may be encouraged to try them. Nutritious dishes which can be prepared with limited cooking facilities may appeal when work or tiredness gives less time or inclination for cooking.

(c) TOBACCO, ALCOHOL AND DRUGS

There can be resistance to discussing the subjects of alcohol and tobacco. Clients can feel they are being 'nagged' and nobody likes that.

Many smokers are aware that medical authorities believe smoking can harm the fetus, but they continue to smoke. The reasons given may be complex, ranging from: 'I don't believe it, my friend had a healthy baby and smoked forty a day', 'It's the only pleasure I get', 'I can't give up, I've tried', to 'I do wish people would stop telling me what I ought to do'. The most appropriate attitude for the antenatal teacher is supportive and non-judgemental. It is well known that smokers produce smaller babies, the effect of nicotine on fetal blood flow has been demonstrated,[4] and recent research has shown a decrease of maternal hormones which may explain some observed adverse effects of smoking in pregnancy.[5] Stopping smoking before sixteen weeks is best, but there is evidence that stopping later still has benefits.[6] Can you offer any concrete help? Find out what is available in your area. Possible support may include: individual counselling, smoking clinic or self-help through peer group support.

Pregnancy

Inducing guilt is neither productive or kind and it may increase stress.

Alcohol consumed by a mother in large quantities will harm a fetus.[7] With present knowledge it is not possible to give an absolute safe limit of alcohol consumption in pregnancy, but the advice to keep to two or three measures per week, if she cannot abstain, is reasonable. It would be cruel to so frighten a woman that she spent the rest of her pregnancy worrying about the effects of one party or moderate consumption in early pregnancy. Ask your clients if they know what constitutes a 'measure' or 'standard drink'? It is commonly believed that spirits are more harmful than beer, whereas a pint of ordinary beer or lager contains twice as much alcohol as a single measure of whisky, and a pint of strong beer or lager can contain five standard drinks. One standard drink contains about 10 grams of alcohol.[8]

When discussing drugs, words and their different meanings and connotations are important. 'Drugs' to you may mean any chemical administered for medicinal or other reasons. To the lay person 'drugs' usually mean heroin, cocaine or another drug of addiction. So if you say 'taking drugs in pregnancy can harm your baby', they may feel that does not apply to them, not considering what they buy from the chemist as a 'drug'. The word 'medicine' may have more relevance. Taking medicines during pregnancy does worry many women and it is helpful to give them clear guidelines to follow. Liaise with other midwives and doctors so the mothers do not receive conflicting advice. If a mother is told by one person that it is safe to take paracetamol for relief of headache or cold symptoms and then another says 'do not take any medicines in pregnancy not directly prescribed', this can cause confusion and destroy trust in those caring for her.[9] Helping those women who are addicted to hard drugs is a specialized field and not likely to form part of regular antenatal classes. You should, however, know where to refer her if such a client presents herself at your classes.

Pregnancy

(d) EXERCISE AND PHYSICAL COMFORT

It is useful to discuss the reasons for the many changes and symptoms which occur in pregnancy apart from increasing girth. This should include the hormonal changes which cause not only nausea but breast discomfort, gastric reflux, relaxed ligaments, varicose veins, frequency of micturition, haemorrhoids and constipation. The increasing size of the uterus can cause discomfort through stretching uterine ligaments, costal margin pain and dyspnoea. Sometimes dismissed as the 'minor disorders of pregnancy', they deserve attention because with the correct advice each woman can minimize the distress caused by these symptoms. Breast discomfort may be reduced by wearing a comfortable, well-supporting bra; however, in a minority breast sensitivity remains a problem throughout pregnancy. Nausea can often be relieved by eating something dry before rising in the morning, and leaping out of bed quickly is not advisable. Separating eating and drinking by a short period may also help. When gastric reflux is a problem, a change of eating habits to small, frequent, blander meals may help, together with attention to position, remaining upright for at least half-an-hour after meals. Sleeping propped up on several pillows or raising the head of the bed on two bricks may also relieve the discomfort. Constipation should be avoidable with a suitable diet, although iron tablets may cause extra problems to some women.

An obstetric physiotherapist is the obvious person to advise on the musculo-skeletal aspects, but you may not have the services of a physiotherapist with this particular expertise. Calf cramp can be troublesome, dorsiflexion of the foot is the answer to both avoidance (stretching in that position) and relief (active or passive stretching of the calf muscle). Physical fitness is as desirable in pregnancy as at any other time in life. Labour and motherhood are hard work and it seems sensible to be prepared. When considering exercise in

Pregnancy

pregnancy strain should be avoided, but exercise to which an individual is accustomed may be continued as long as it is comfortable.[10] Those who normally exercise little can be encouraged to walk or perhaps swim. Emphasis on getting fit for labour may induce some to take up a new exercise or sport. Caution should be used or strain may result through lack of understanding by client or sports coach. Yoga can be beneficial in increasing suppleness and body awareness, but some postures are unsuitable in pregnancy and anyone teaching yoga to pregnant women must be aware of this.[11]

Women may anticipate trying alternative positions in labour, such as squatting. Few westerners are used to this position and will need to practise squatting over a period of time before they are comfortable. Exercises which improve the tone in those muscles under special strain at this time, such as abdomen and pelvic floor, will be beneficial not only now, but also after birth. Abdominal muscle strengthening exercises must put no strain on the back, for example, double leg raising must never be attempted.[12]

Pelvic floor exercises are arguably the most important exercises a woman can do. Much discomfort and distress caused by incompetent pelvic floor muscles in many women, young and old, may be avoided by correct teaching in the antenatal period. Exercising pelvic floor muscles can relieve discomfort when pressure is experienced in later pregnancy and stress incontinence can be avoided if the client is taught to brace her pelvic floor when coughing or sneezing. Awareness of and the ability to control the pelvic floor can aid delivery. After birth, pain and swelling can be eased and the return to full recovery speeded, including return to a satisfactory sex life. There is no point in being coy when teaching pelvic floor exercises. Telling a mother to 'tighten her bottom' may merely produce a contraction in her buttocks. Using images she can relate to will be more effective, for example, 'imagine you are desperate to use the toilet and there is a queue.' Many women are asked to

Pregnancy

produce mid-stream specimens of urine which they can do without difficulty. You can build on this skill to develop awareness of the pelvic floor.[13] To attain good muscle tone, fifty is a reasonable number of pelvic floor contractions per day antenatally, but pelvic floor muscles fatigue quickly, so four tightenings at a time are enough.

Good posture can be taught and maintained better in pregnancy by encouraging mothers to 'grow tall' and 'tuck your tail bone under', rather than instructions to 'stand straight and pull your shoulders back'. Tilting the pelvis back not only aids back comfort but also lessens strain on abdominal muscles. Good posture can also have a beneficial effect on morale. 'Standing tall' can help to minimize the discomfort caused by the large uterus pushing the ribs out sideways. If actual pain occurs from this cause, stretching sideways away from the pain may help. It is necessary to be conscious of correct posture not only when standing but also when sitting and working. Good positions in lying can also greatly aid comfort.[14] Lifting techniques are taught to nurses and midwives, and you should pass on these skills to your clients.

The usual positions of sitting, resting and sleeping may become uncomfortable in pregnancy and mothers can be encouraged to discover alternatives: for example, sitting astride an armless chair and leaning on a cushion on the chairback or lying in the 'recovery position' with a pillow supporting the top leg.

A pregnant mother's back is vulnerable; hormonal changes will have relaxed the ligaments by sixteen weeks' gestation, and the growing fetus causes postural adjustments and the abdominal supports are weakened. The ligaments will not return to normal until four to five months after birth, so mothers need advice not only on posture and lifting in pregnancy, but also on back care after birth. This can include buying suitable prams and choosing sensible positions for changing baby's nappy. The maximum effect of relaxed

Pregnancy

ligaments will be experienced at thirty-eight weeks' gestation by mothers expecting their second baby[15] and as these women may well have a toddler to care for, they need to be extra vigilant in avoiding strain. Back pain in pregnancy should not be ignored and accepted as inevitable. Physiotherapy can often give relief. Specific exercises or a sacro-iliac support may be effective.[16] Midwives do not have the skills to diagnose or treat back pain but they can ensure mothers know they can ask for help and that appropriate referrals are made. Carpal tunnel syndrome and pain due to pubic diastasis are two other conditions for which physiotherapists can offer assistance.[17]

We may only be able to offer sympathy and reassurance about some of the aches and pains of pregnancy, but we can ensure everything possible has been done. The 'minor problems of pregnancy' may not seem so 'minor' when you are suffering.

It is sometimes difficult to be comfortable travelling in a car wearing a seat belt in the later stages of pregnancy. Mothers may ask if they can legally dispense with their seat belts. Pregnancy is not normally sufficient reason to do so, although exemption is possible with a doctor's certificate stating that the wearing of seat belts is medically inadvisable.[18] An Australian study showed seat belts as a cause of placental abruptions in accidents; lap-only belts were more dangerous than lap and diagonal belts. However, more maternal deaths occurred when seat belts were not worn.[19] Advice could be given to mothers to report any sharp deceleration incident to her obstetrician, even when no injury was apparent.

(e) EMOTIONS AND SEX IN PREGNANCY

A woman's emotions in pregnancy can be labile and she may be more able to cope with this if she understands how normal this is. Reading women's accounts of their feelings during pregnancy and after can be illuminating, especially if you have not experienced pregnancy yourself.[20,21] Professional

Pregnancy

women used to responsibility may find themselves unable to make decisions as they used to; many women become forgetful and find themselves weeping for trivial reasons. Even in a wanted pregnancy, feelings of ambivalence or even resentment are not uncommon. An acknowledgement of these feelings and an opportunity to discuss them can be a great relief. Women may feel happy about giving up work or lonely and bored at home, alone. They may have weird, vivid dreams. They may feel unattractive and worry about the reaction of their boyfriend or husband to their changing shape. The relationship with him will undergo a change, as will their inclination for lovemaking (see Chapter 6).

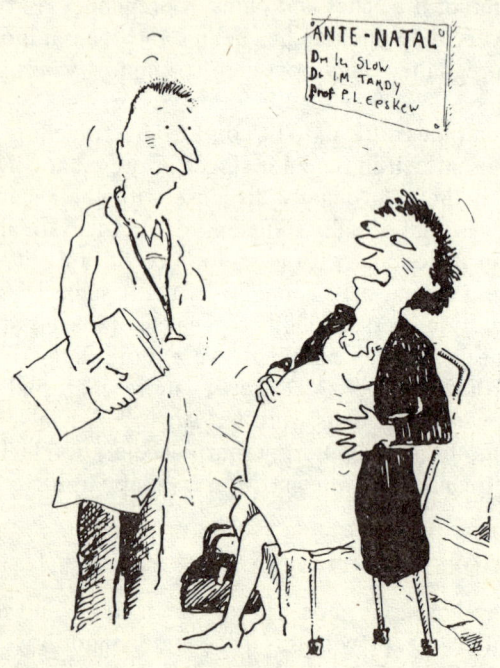

While I've been sat here the dinner's burnt, the cat's died, and my old man's run off with the postman. And *you* talk to *me* about blood pressure.'

Pregnancy

(f) ANTENATAL CARE

Antenatal care should ideally be a team effort between the mother (or couple) and those caring for her. She is after all a person responsible for her life and her co-operation is needed to ensure the best possible outcome. Antenatal clinic visits, unfortunately, are sometimes seen by the women as a tedious waste of time: 'Two hours wait and two minutes with the doctor'. Maybe it is not like that in your hospital. Think about the ways that you can help your clients not only to understand what we are trying to do in antenatal care, but how they can get the best out of their visits. For example, if the mother is shy and the doctor always seems rushed, so that questions go unanswered and maybe unasked, you could suggest that she writes her questions down before she goes to the clinic. The doctor saying 'all is well' may not reassure the mother. We often talk of informed choice; why not also informed reassurance? Doctors and midwives often use terms or say things in ways which confuse and frighten women, even when the intention is the opposite. A doctor may say 'You've a good big baby there', and the woman may spend the next week worrying if it will be too big to come out normally. You cannot prepare women for everything that might be said to them, but you can help them to acquire the confidence to ask if they are puzzled. The advice you can give in class cannot always be specific enough for every client, and if their care is to be of the highest quality they need to be able to communicate with the person directly in charge of their care. In class you can reinforce the information and advice given to them in clinic about the routine tests and observations. If co-operation cards are used this can be a useful starting point for discussion, explaining the terms used and the reasons for tests and observations carried out. Are you up to date with the latest procedures at your local hospitals? If research projects are in progress the staff involved are often very pleased to talk to interested colleagues. You could

Pregnancy

discuss the purposes of ultrasound scanning. This procedure can give reassurance and pleasure to some, but others are worried that there will be possible ill effects on the fetus.[22,23]

Exposure to hazards could be discussed. Avoiding unnecessary exposure to any infections is sensible, without restricting normal life too much. Clients could be encouraged to report exposure to any serious or unusual illness to their doctor. Hopefully they are protected against rubella and should be aware if they are not. Toxoplasmosis is one infection they may be exposed to without their knowledge and it would be sensible to eat meat that had been well cooked and to avoid any contact with cat faeces as may happen if they clean the litter tray of a pet cat.[24,25] Particular food contamination hazards may become apparent from time to time.[26] As a pregnant woman and her fetus are among the more vulnerable members of society she should be given information and advice about food hygiene.

Women may be concerned about potential hazards at work or in the general environment. Studies have attempted to assess the risk to the fetus.[27,28] But the picture is far from clear. It may be beyond the power of an individual to avoid all hazards in this increasingly technological world, but a mother whose work brings her into contact with industrial chemicals should certainly question their safety with her Health and Safety representative. Travel in pregnancy may be discussed. Women must balance their need or desire to travel with potential risks. Specific advice should be sought about exposure to infections likely to be encountered and immunization during pregnancy. The effects of high altitude, and this can include airliner cabin pressure, may be significant to some women, for example those suffering from sickle cell disease or anaemia.[29] If common sense is used, travel during pregnancy should not be a problem for most women.

There are so many things that worry pregnant women that it is impossible for one teacher to cover all eventualities: therefore it is important to give opportunities for worries to

Pregnancy

be voiced. Many women say: 'This may be a silly question but . . .'. They need to feel safe enough to ask that 'silly question'. It probably isn't silly and it is important to them.

(g) LAYETTE AND BABY EQUIPMENT

It is often a complaint about antenatal classes that layette is discussed after most people have already completed their shopping. You need to think about at what stage of pregnancy you will cover this. Think about how a mother decides what she needs to buy for her baby. Lists of clothes and equipment are often produced by those with a commercial interest and mothers can be persuaded to spend more than they need or can afford. Encourage them to look critically at a list and decide how many of the things they could do without. When considering the number of first-size clothes, ask them how long they think an average-sized baby would be likely to fit into them and also how quickly they will be able to get them washed and dried. Ask them to reflect on how long a baby may sleep in a crib. Perhaps the baby could go into a drop-side cot from birth, then a crib would be unnecessary. Encourage them to think about why they need particular items rather than providing them with a list of essentials. It may be helpful to acknowledge the superstition of 'tempting fate' if too much or indeed any baby equipment is purchased before the birth. Those who believe this will not then feel odd or abnormal. Gifts may come from friends and relatives, so mothers could wait and see what they do not provide. Ask them to think about second-hand equipment. Local newspapers and health clinic notice boards are two possible sources; do you know of any other local ones?

Teaching mothers to be aware of good design and safety factors will be useful. Suggest ways of looking at equipment so they buy that which is safe and good value for money. You could explain the function of the British Standards Institution and the British Electrotechnical Board. Friends and

Pregnancy

relatives can be a source of information about good and bad equipment. Consumer research magazines, radio and television programmes give useful information. Magazines aimed at parents of young children often conduct consumer research, giving a broader view of the range of equipment. No antenatal teacher can be up to date on every piece of equipment on the market, but if you teach them how to judge, you help them to make sensible choices. Buying well-designed equipment can affect their health; a pram, nappy-changing table or baby bath that causes them to work with a bent back can cause backache. A pram handle should be at a height which enables a mother to push it with her forearms horizontal; any lower and she will bend forward.

(h) SAFETY IN THE HOME

It may seem too early to encourage clients to think about safety beyond the baby stage, but it is sensible to cultivate an awareness of safety from the beginning. Homes are dangerous places and children can so easily get into trouble. Ask clients to think about what hazards a crawling baby would face in their homes. Open fires, boiling saucepans on cookers, stairs and medicines are some obvious hazards in the home, but what else may be dangerous? What temperature does the outside of the oven door reach during cooking? Does the kettle flex trail over the edge of the work surface? Where are the cleaning materials kept? Almost every substance to be found in a home has been swallowed by a child at some time somewhere. Child-resistant catches can be fitted to drawers and cupboards. Every child goes through the stage of putting everything into his mouth. House plants are not meant to be eaten and may be poisonous.[30] A crawling baby's eye view of a home can reveal many potential hazards. Patio or other glass doors can be a hazard; if it is not safety glass a transparent sticky-backed film can be applied to prevent sharp splinters being showered around if it

Pregnancy

is broken. Ask them to think about what provisions should be made if there are pets. Even the best loved animal cannot be completely trusted alone with a baby. Cat nets to fit cots and prams are a necessary safeguard. Fleas and worms can infest a crawling baby.

(i) CAR SAFETY

The safety of babies in cars has received much attention in recent years and the consensus of opinion is that the safest method of transport for a baby is a specifically designed infant carrier.[31,32] All the models marketed in this country reach the required safety standards. A carry cot, even when correctly harnessed, does not give as good protection in an accident. In many parts of the country there are schemes which loan or sell infant carriers at a reduced price. You may find your local road safety officer willing to talk to your clients.

(j) RIGHTS AND BENEFITS

Do you know the rights of pregnant working women? Do you know the basic rules applying to a mother's receipt of benefits during her pregnancy and afterwards? The DHSS supplies leaflets for distribution and more comprehensive booklets explaining the rules.[33,34] Sometimes a mother's entitlement may not be clear and she may need to apply for an appointment at a DHSS office. She may be more successful in her claim if she has a good knowledge of the possibilties. Sources of help are Maternity Alliance, The National Council for Civil Liberties[35] and The Association for the Improvement of Maternity Services (see Appendix 1).

(k) ....

Can you think of anything else clients may need or want to know?

Pregnancy

4 How Will You Teach?

This chapter has covered a wide range of subjects which will probably be taught at different sessions. Some subjects may require a greater input of factual information from you, such as fetal development, travel safety and rights and benefits. Other topics, for example, emotions, need more opportunity for discussion. In any topic, if you can assess clients' present knowledge and opinions by encouraging them to talk and ask questions, you can then build on what they know. Exercises and positions for comfort are obviously most easily taught and learnt by demonstration and practice.

5 What Aids Will You Use?

Slides or a video are useful for portraying fetal development, and can help to make the fetus seem more real.[36,37] The book *Being Born* contains many of Lennart Nilsson's photographs of fetal life.[38] Sometimes questions are raised about how such photographs are obtained; clients may want reassurance that they are not looking at dead babies.

Slides or posters could be used to illustrate nutrition: real food may have more impact but would be difficult and costly to organize. Leaflets are useful to reinforce your teaching and provide a reminder for clients to retain (see below).

A sample layette and some items of baby equipment are useful. It is not necessary to have all essential items; an incomplete display can be a good starting point for discussion. Local shops may be prepared to provide items for you to show to mothers.

Two short videos illustrating safety in the home and safety in cars are available.[39]

Videos to trigger discussion on various aspects of pregnancy may be useful.[40]

Pregnancy

6   Trigger Questions For Discussion

What physical changes have you noticed since you became pregnant?
What changes have you noticed in your emotions since your pregnancy began?
Can you tell us about any 'old wives' tales' of pregnancy that you have heard?
Have there been any changes or feelings that have surprised you?
Your baby has started, or soon will start to kick you. Do you know what else he or she can do inside you?
What changes do you think you should make in your diet when you are pregnant?
What do you feel about drinking alcohol while you are pregnant?
What exercise do you enjoy?
What exercise do you think is suitable for you while you are pregnant?
What did you feel when you saw your baby on the ultrasound machine?
Have you anything written on your co-operation card that you do not understand?
What clothes or equipment have you bought for your baby?
Can you think of anything in your home that might be a danger to a crawling baby?
What do you know of safe ways for a baby to travel in a car?
How do you think pets may react to a new baby in the house?

7   How Will You Know When You Have Achieved Your Aims And Objectives?

You cannot know if a client will change her diet or stop smoking, but if she shows a willingness to do so in discussion you will have achieved what is possible to measure at that

Pregnancy

point. She can demonstrate exercises and different positions. In the course of discussion you can ask her to recall essential factors in choosing equipment or organizing her home. You are not running an examination course and it is not possible to check all learning thoroughly, but you will be able to make an estimate of the effectiveness of your teaching.

Suggested Leaflets

From Health Education Authority:

A Guide to Healthy Eating.
That's the Limit: A Guide to Sensible Drinking.
How to Stop Smoking for You and Your Baby.

Eat Better for Less. From: Community Dietitian, Health Education Service, Harness House, Basingstoke District Hospital, Basingstoke, RG24 9NB.

From the Community Dietitians, Charing Cross Hospital, Fulham Palace Road, London W6:

Food for a Healthy Life – Without Cooking.
Food for a Healthy Life – In a Bed-Sit.

Exercise leaflets from Milupa Educational Services:

Care of Your Body in Pregnancy.
The Birth.
Postnatal Exercises and Advice.

Safety leaflets from the Child Accident Prevention Trust:

Keep Your Baby Safe: A Guide to Safe Nursery Equipment.
Keep Them Safe: A Guide to Child Safety Equipment.

Pregnancy

First Ride Safe Ride: Keeping Your Baby Safe in the Car.

Look After Your Child in the Car. Department of Transport.
Your Home is Dangerous. RoSPA.
It CAN Happen to You. Some hints on home safety. Association of British Insurers.
Babies and Benefits. A guide to benefits for expectant and new mothers. DHSS leaflet FB8.

From Maternity Alliance:

Getting Fit for Pregnancy.
Pregnant at Work.
Money for Mothers and Babies.

For addresses see Appendix 1.

References

1 Olds, C. (1985), 'Fetal response to music', *Midwives Chronicle*, vol. 98, no. 1170, July, pp. 202–3.
2 Truswell, A. S. (1985), 'Nutrition for pregnancy', *British Medical Journal*, vol. 291, 27 July, pp. 263–6.
3 *Asians in Britain. A Study of Their Dietary Patterns in Relation to Their Cultural and Religious Backgrounds* (1976), Van den Berghs and Jurgens Ltd., Public Relations Department, Sussex House, Civic Way, Burgess Hill, Sussex, RH15 9AW.
4 Lindblad, A., Maršál, K. and Andersson, K-E. (1988), 'Effect of nicotine on human blood flow', *Obstetrics and Gynaecology*, vol. 72, no. 3, part 1, September, pp. 371–81.
5 Bernstein, L., Pike, M. C., Lobo, R. A., Depue, R. H., Ross, R. K. and Henderson, B. E. (1989), 'Cigarette smoking in pregnancy results in marked decrease in maternal hCG and oestradiol levels', *British Journal of Obstetrics and Gynaecology*, vol. 96, January, pp. 92–6.
6 MacArthur, C. and Knox, E. G. (1988), 'Smoking in pregnancy: effects of stopping at different stages', *British Journal of Obstetrics and Gynaecology*, vol. 95, June, pp. 551–5.
7 Rosett, H. L., Weiner, L., Lee, A., Zuckerman, B., Dooling, E. and Oppenheimer, E. (1983), 'Patterns of alcohol consumption and fetal

development', *Obstetrics and Gynaecology*, vol. 61, no. 5, May, pp. 539–46.

8 (1986), *Alcohol and Smoking. A Guide for Midwives*, London Health Education Council.

9 Hawkins, D. F. Ed. (1987), *Drugs and Pregnancy*, Churchill Livingstone, Edinburgh.

10 Jackson, P. (1986), 'Diary of a Pregnant Woman', *Nursing*, vol. 3, no. 1, pp. 24–5.

11 Noble, E. (1978), *Essential Exercises for the Childbearing Year*, John Murray, London, pp. 15–19.

12 Ibid., pp. 63–81.

13 Ibid., pp. 20–44.

14 Ibid., pp. 82–120.

15 Polden, M. (1987), 'Pain relief in obstetrics and gynaecology'. In: *Pain: Management and Control in Physiotherapy*, Wells, P. E., Frampton, V. and Bowsher, D. (eds), Heinemann, London, p. 283.

16 Ibid., pp. 284–8.

17 Ibid., pp. 289–90.

18 Street, H. (1984), Cons. Ed, *You and Your Rights. An A to Z Guide to the Law*. Reader's Digest, London, p. 649.

19 Chetcuti, P. and Levene, M. I. (1987), 'Seat belts: a potential hazard to the fetus', *Journal of Perinatal Medicine*, vol. 15, p. 207.

20 Breen, D. (1981), *Talking with Mothers*, Jill Norman, London.

21 Oakley, A. (1979), *From Here to Maternity, Becoming a Mother*, Penguin, Harmondsworth.

22 Meire, H. B. (1987), 'The safety of diagnostic ultrasound', *British Journal of Obstetrics and Gynaecology*, vol. 94, December, pp. 1121–2.

23 (1985), 'Ultrasound in pregnancy: should it be routine?', *Drug and Therapeutics Bulletin*, vol. 23, no. 15, July 29, pp. 57–60.

24 Charles, D. and Larsen, B. (1984), 'Protozoal, fungal and bacterial infections'. In: *Medical and Surgical Problems in Obstetrics*, Brudenell, M. and Wilds, P. L. (eds), Wright, Bristol, pp. 233–5.

25 Butler, V. (1983), 'Toxoplasmosis', *Midwives Chronicle*, vol. 96, no. 1140, January, p. 17.

26 Holmes, S. (1989), 'Careful food handling reduces the risk of *Listeria*', *The Professional Nurse*, vol. 4, no. 7, April, pp. 322–4.

27 Longo, L. D. (1980), 'Environmental pollution and pregnancy: risks and uncertainties for the fetus and infant', *American Journal of Obstetrics and Gynaecology*, vol. 137, no. 2, pp. 162–73.

28 Lee, W. R. (1985), 'Working with visual display units'. *British Medical Journal*, vol. 291, 12 October, pp. 989–91.

29 Barry, M. and Bia, F. (1989), 'Pregnancy and travel', *Journal of American Medical Association*, vol. 261, no. 5, 3 February, pp. 728–31.

Pregnancy

30 Asher, J. (1988), *Keep Your Baby Safe. A Guide to the Prevention and Treatment of Accidents and Medical Emergencies in Babies and Children up to Three*, Penguin, Harmondsworth, pp. 43–5.

31 Avery, G. and Avery, P. (1987), 'Child safety in cars', *Maternal and Child Health*, vol. 12, no. 10, October, pp. 288–94.

32 Trezise, V. (1988), 'The need for restraint', *Midwives Chronicle*, vol. 101, no. 1203, April, pp. 117–19.

33 *Employers' Guide to Statutory Maternity Pay*, DHSS leaflet NI. 257.

34 *Maternity Benefits. A Technical Guide*, DHSS leaflet NI. 17A.

35 Coussins, J., Durward, L. and Evans, R. (1987), *Maternity Rights at Work*, National Council for Civil Liberties, Women's Rights Unit, NCCL, 21 Tabard Street, London, SE1 4LA.

36 *Having a Baby*, Video, BBC Enterprises.

37 *The Development of the Fetus*. Slides from Farleys.

38 Kitzinger, K. and Nilsson, L. (1986), *Being Born*, Dorling Kindersley, London.

39 *First Ride, Safe Ride: Keeping Baby Safe in the Car* and *Keep Them Safe*, Child Accident Prevention Trust, 28 Portland Place, London, W1N 4DE.

40 *Testing and Guiding* and *Myths*, Farleys Trigger Films/Videos.

Further Reading

Cornford-Wood, L. J. (1986), 'Normal Pregnancy', *Nursing*, vol. 3, no. 1, January, pp. 2–7.

Dale, B. and Roeber, J. (1982), *Exercises for Childbirth*, Century, London.

Ellis, C. E. G. (1986), 'The assessment of fetal well-being', *Nursing*, vol. 3, no. 1, January, pp. 8–12.

Henley, A. (1979), *Asian Patients in Hospital and at Home*, King Edward's Hospital Fund for London, pp. 75–81.

Huws, U. (1987), *VDU Hazards Handbook. A Worker's Guide to the Effects of New Technology*, London Hazards Centre, Third Floor, Headland House, 308 Gray's Inn Road, London WC1X 8DS.

Jamieson, L. (1986), 'Education for Parenthood', *Nursing*, vol. 3, no. 1, January, pp. 13–16.

Kohner, N. (1984), *Pregnancy Book. A Guide to Becoming Pregnant, Being Pregnant and Caring for Your Newborn Baby*, Health Education Council, London.

Kohner, N. (1988), *Having a Baby*, BBC Publications, London.

Oakley, A. (1986), *The Captured Womb. A History of the Medical Care of Pregnant Women*, Basil Blackwell, Oxford.

Prince, J. and Adams, M. E. (1987), *The Psychology of Childbirth. An*

Pregnancy

Introduction for Mothers and Midwives, 2nd edn, Churchill Livingstone, Edinburgh.

Smith, V.A. (1986), 'High risk and complicated pregnancy', *Nursing*, vol. 3, no. 1, January, pp. 20–3.

Stearn, M. (1986), 'Social and psychological aspects of pregnancy', *Nursing*, vol. 3, no. 1, January, pp. 17–19.

Target, G. (1986), *How to Stop Smoking*, Sheldon, London.

Religions and Cultures. A Guide to Patients' Beliefs and Customs for Health Service Staff (1978), Lothian Community Relations Council, 12a Forth Street, Edinburgh, EH1 3LH (Tel: 031-556-0441).

6
Relaxation and Breathing for Labour

The physical preparation is often undertaken by an obstetric physiotherapist, but you may be expected to teach these subjects. Relaxation is a life skill useful to us all. If you have not already done so, learn a technique yourself. You will be more able to teach relaxation if you understand how your chosen method works. Breathing cannot be taught in isolation and in the teaching situation must be linked to all the other considerations pertaining to labour (see Chapter 7). You will be teaching skills; think about how you expect your clients to use those skills.

1 What Are Your Aims?

Clients will be able to:

Minimize the amount of pain relief (drugs) they will require in labour.
As far as possible remain in control of their labours.
Make the best use of their energy resources in labour.
Increase their self-reliance.
Increase body awareness.
Or . . .?

Having your aims in mind,

Relaxation and Breathing for Labour

2 What Are Your Objectives?

At the end of the session the mother will be able to:

Demonstrate recognition of the need for relaxation.
Relax.
Recall the breathing patterns to be used in labour.
Demonstrate confidence in her ability to cope with labour.
Show increased body awareness.
Or . . .?

3 What Will You Teach?

(a) CHOICE OF RELAXATION METHOD

The ability to relax is useful not only for labour, but also for all those occasions when we may be stressed; when the baby is screaming but won't feed, when you are in a traffic jam and late for work, just before the first teaching session with a new group. These are times when we need a quick method to reduce tension and allow us to continue with our lives in a happier, more efficient and less tiring way. Regular sessions where an attempt is made to achieve a deeper physical and mental relaxation are also beneficial.

If you are a member of a team of antenatal teachers, there will probably be an accepted method and it is logical that all are teaching the same technique. If, however, you have to decide which method to use, consider the alternatives; but whichever method you use, try it for yourself and know that it works before you attempt to teach. Some methods have very old origins, such as yoga, which uses posture and awareness of breathing to achieve a conscious relaxation of mind and body.[1] Some methods use similar techniques to those which form the basis of meditation, teaching 'mindfulness' of breathing and/or concentration on a thought, object or

Relaxation and Breathing for Labour

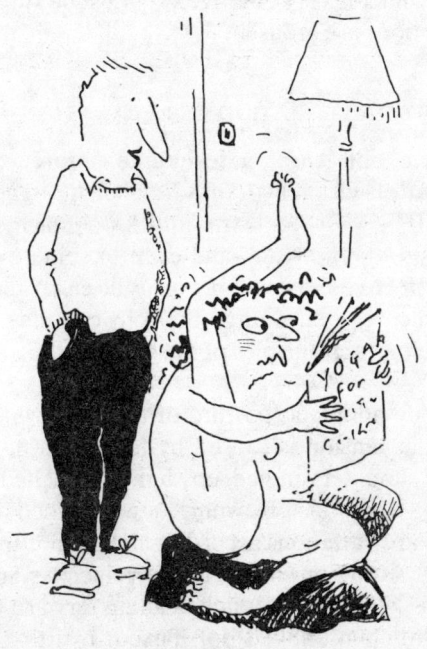

'Relaxing, dear?'

sound.[2] Some use exercises as a preliminary to relaxation.[3] Some seek to induce relaxation by directing the thoughts to various parts of the body, relaxing each in turn.[4] Alternatively, the client is taught a pattern of tensing then relaxing muscles, progressively relaxing different parts of the body.[5] Touch can be used; self-massage such as gently kneading neck muscles or smoothing the forehead can aid relaxation.[6] A partner can use touch, gently laying a hand on the part of the body on which the woman is concentrating. This could be practised between mothers in a class. If you are teaching couples then touch can be a pleasant and useful part of the relaxation technique.[7] A teacher should be aware of possible inhibitions which may cause tension instead of relaxation.

Relaxation and Breathing for Labour

Physical contact is very emotive; we must be sure that appropriate emotions are aroused.

(b) THE MITCHELL METHOD OF RELAXATION

If you have not learnt a technique before, the Mitchell Method of Relaxation by Laura Mitchell has much to recommend it. It is easy to learn, quick to teach and can be practised sitting and lying, and even to some extent, standing. It is effective in producing a result easily discernible by clients, which can encourage them to continue to practise. The physiological principles of this method are:

1   The body adopts a 'posture of tension', which is similar whether that tension is caused by fear, pain or anger. This posture is shoulders pulled up, hands clenched, arms held close to the body, face frowning, jaw clenched, teeth grinding. There are variations according to whether the individual is standing, sitting or lying, but the principles are the same. The body is held rigid, possibly leaning forward, the legs are tense, slightly bent, ankles dorsiflexed. If sitting the legs are crossed, or even entwined.
2   Reciprocal relaxation. For each group of muscles that contracts to perform a movement or maintain a position, the opposing group must relax. Try it: with your palm facing upwards bend your arm to make a right angle at the elbow. Palpate your biceps muscle: it is hard, contracted; now palpate your loose triceps below: feel the difference?

The method uses these principles in a series of small movements designed to relax those muscles which contract in the posture of tension and put the joints into a position of ease and comfort. The method teaches consciousness of joint position and skin pressure not muscle tension awareness, since this is not registered in the upper brain.[8]

Each self-order initiates a movement which works a group

of muscles that oppose part of the tension posture. The first order is 'pull your shoulders towards your feet'. The next instruction is 'stop', not 'relax' but stop doing the movement. The client is then invited to feel the new position of the shoulders downwards. The programme continues with orders for movements to produce relaxation in each group of muscles which contract in the posture of tension.

The following extract is from *Simple Relaxation*, Laura Mitchell,[9] pages 60–2.

CHECK LIST OF ORDERS
ARMS
Shoulders
Order: Pull your shoulders towards your feet. STOP
Result: Feel your shoulders are further away from your ears. Your neck may feel longer.
Elbows
Order: Elbows out and open. STOP
Result: Feel your upper arms away from your body and the wide angle at your elbows. The weight of both arms should be resting on the floor, chair arms or pillow.
Hands
Order: Fingers and thumbs long and supported. STOP
Result: Feel your fingers and thumbs stretched out, separated, and touching support, nails on top. Especially feel your heavy thumbs.
LEGS
Hips
Order: Turn your hips outwards. STOP
Result: Feel your thighs rolled outwards. Kneecaps face outwards.
Knees
Order: Move slightly until comfortable if you wish. STOP
Result: Feel the resulting comfort in your knees.

Relaxation and Breathing for Labour

Feet
Order: Push your feet away from your face, bending at the ankle. STOP
Result: Feel your heavy dangling feet.
BODY
Order: Push your body into the support. STOP
Result: Feel the contact of your body on the support.
HEAD
Order: Push your head into the support. STOP
Result: Feel the contact of your head on the support or pressure on the pillow.
BREATHING
Choose the rate but try to keep it slow. Choose placing in routine before or after body and head, or when you feel your breathing rate slowing down. *Breathe in gently*. Expand the area in front above the waist, and between the angles of the rib cage, and raise your lower ribs upwards and outwards like the wings of a bird. Then *breathe out gently*. Feel your ribs fall downwards and inwards. Repeat once or at most twice.
FACE
Jaw
Order: Drag your jaw downwards. STOP
Result: Feel your separated teeth, heavy jaw, and soft lips gently touching each other.
Tongue
Order: Press your tongue downwards in your mouth. STOP
Result: Feel your tongue loose and slack gullet.
Eyes
Order: Close your eyes. STOP
Result: Feel your upper lids resting gently over your eyes, without any screwing up around the eyes. Enjoy the darkness.
Forehead
Order: Begin above eyebrows and think of smoothing gently up into your hair, over the top of your head and down the back of your neck. STOP

Relaxation and Breathing for Labour

Result: Feel your hair move in the same direction.
MIND
Order: Either repeat the above sequence around the body, possibly more quickly. Or choose some subject which you will enjoy thinking about, and which has a sequence (song, prayer, poem, multiplication table, etc.). Or relive some past personal happy occasion. Let the mind play over these thoughts effortlessly, just to keep it occupied.
RETURN TO FULL ACTIVITY
Always stretch limbs and body in all directions and yawn. Do not hurry. Sit up slowly and wait a minute or two before standing up.

In order to have a complete understanding of this method and why and how it works, anyone teaching it is advised to read the whole book. A cassette of the Mitchell Method of Relaxation is available.[10]

(b) MENTAL RELAXATION

Relaxation of the body is perhaps easier to achieve than relaxation of the mind. The mind is wilful and it takes a firm but gentle discipline to quieten it. Although some methods teach 'emptying the mind', it is difficult without considerable practice for the mind to concentrate on nothing, to be completely still. At first it is useful to concentrate on one object, picture or pattern, or sound either in reality or in the mind. Every time the mind wanders it is brought back to dwell on the chosen subject. If concentrating on one thing proves difficult then a sequence can be followed, provided this does not stimulate thoughts which go off at a tangent, for example, mentally reciting a poem or visualizing a familiar walk. Care should be taken that the chosen subject does not itself cause the start of a chain of thoughts which activate the brain. It is no good a client imagining that she is lying on a beach in the sun if that makes her think of writing postcards

Relaxation and Breathing for Labour

on the beach last holiday and how mother-in-law was upset because we didn't send her a postcard and she's coming to lunch on Sunday and what am I going to cook! A teacher can make suggestions for a suitable subjects but should encourage clients to choose for themselves.

(d) BREATHING IN RELAXATION

Teaching clients to be aware of their breathing can aid the relaxation process but imposing the rate is not helpful. It can be suggested they breathe a little slower than normal and possibly pause slightly after the outbreath at first, then merely to be aware of the natural slowing of respiration that occurs during relaxation. Deep relaxation not only decreases the rate of breathing, but also decreases the heart rate and reduces the body's consumption of oxygen.[11] A sudden return to an upright posture can cause giddiness. When you wish to terminate the relaxation session encourage them to stretch first and ensure that they resume activity slowly and gently.

(e) REASONS FOR TEACHING BREATHING FOR LABOUR

You will not of course teach people to breathe, we all know how to do that. Many of us, however, do not use our full lung capacity, as singers, actors and musicians are taught to do. Antenatal classes may be a good opportunity to teach efficient use of the lungs. This can be achieved by teaching abdominal or diaphragmatic breathing.[12] In this type of breathing, during inspiration the abdominal wall expands, the ribs move upwards and outwards as the diaphragm flattens, allowing the lungs to expand fully. During expiration the reverse movements happen, the ribs move downwards and inwards, the abdomen is firmly flattened as the diaphragm returns to its dome shape, compressing the lungs into the chest cavity and ensuring efficient emptying of the waste

Relaxation and Breathing for Labour

gases. With practice this type of breathing can improve lung function. If practised slowly and at clients' own rate, never forced, giddiness and strain will be prevented. If clients are very unused to such activity very short periods of four or five deep breaths are advisable at first. In later pregnancy when the rising fundus is pushing the ribs out and preventing full movement of the diaphragm, such deep breathing becomes more difficult and it is not the ideal time to teach this for the first time.

Breathing in labour should not be a great conscious effort. Clients can be taught how to modify their breathing in a stressful situation. Why do we need to teach any modification of a natural function? Every midwife will have seen the woman who is not coping well in labour: not only is she very tense but she is breathing with the deep and fast gasping breaths of one who is panic-stricken; she is hyperventilating. Does it really matter if a labouring woman hyperventilates? The abnormally low level of carbon dioxide in the blood which results from hyperventilation produces unpleasant sensations of peripheral numbness and spasm of the hand or foot muscles, and giddiness. This can be frightening for the mother but potentially dangerous for the fetus. Extreme maternal hyperventilation may cause fetal hypoxia, and a fetus who is already compromised may become hypoxic if the mother hyperventilates to a lesser degree.[13] By teaching the skill of appropriate breathing you can extend the armoury of coping strategies which can enable a mother to make efficient use of her energy resources, and maximize her chances of normal and satisfying labour and birth.

(f) CHOICE OF METHOD OF BREATHING IN LABOUR

If you do not already know, find out if there is an accepted method in your hospital or district. Familiarize yourself with that method. If you have to choose which method to teach, consider the alternatives. Some methods teach the client to concentrate on breathing at different levels in the chest, according to the stage of labour reached. Some clients find this complicated and difficult to learn. Upper chest breathing can be a sign of anxiety and tension; it also increases the risk of hyperventilation.[14] If we try to impose on a woman a way of breathing that feels artificial to her, she is likely to find it difficult to learn. She may also find it difficult to remember in labour and tiring to maintain. All methods vary the breathing as contractions increase in intensity. The simplest method of breathing for labour teaches the mother to keep her breathing as slow and low as the intensity of the contractions will allow.

Think about whether you will teach breathing with mouth open or closed. Some teachers prefer breathe in mouth closed, breathe out mouth open. This may not feel comfortable and natural to some women. If breathing in and out with closed lips feels right, then the teacher should not try to impose her own idea. Breathing in with the mouth open does not allow the air to be warmed and moistened in the nose. One result of long periods of energetic mouth breathing is a dry, sore throat.

(g) BREATHING FOR THE FIRST STAGE OF LABOUR

Two important points are the beginning and end of each contraction. Start each contraction with a breath out, then a slow relaxing breath in and out. This gives the woman a well-oxygenated start and calms and focuses the mind for the work ahead. A similar breath at the end of the contraction relaxes her and enables her to make maximum use of the resting periods between contractions.[15]

Breathing should remain calm and the rate kept as slow as feels comfortable to the woman. As the breathing becomes naturally faster with the increasing intensity of the contractions, teaching her to keep the faster breaths shallow helps to avoid hyperventilation. Visualization is useful here. For

Relaxation and Breathing for Labour

example, breathing in a way that will just flicker the flame on an imaginary candle but will not blow it out.

One problem can occur if, for example, because of pethidine a mother dozes through the beginning of a contraction, then wakes suddenly, hit by the full force of a strong contraction and is unable to organize her breathing. Panic breathing – hyperventilating – is likely to ensue. A useful first-aid measure is for her to give one strong blow out, before trying again to get into the desired rhythm. It literally gives her breathing space to collect herself.

It is useful to tell mothers how to deal with the effects of hyperventilation should it occur. The lowered levels of carbon dioxide in the blood need to be returned to normal. Breathing into a paper bag is often suggested as a remedy, but as a bag may not be available on the labour ward, breathing into cupped hands works just as well.

When using Entonox a woman often breathes fairly fast, but in this situation shallow breathing would not enable her to obtain adequate pain relief from the gas. Fairly deep breaths at a normal rate produce the most efficient analgesia.[16]

Maintaining appropriate breathing patterns is often most difficult during the transition stage of labour. The woman may be tired and despondent and feels unable to cope with the contractions at the peak of their intensity. Continuous encouragement, possibly with eye-to-eye contact, is helpful to many mothers. This stage can sometimes be complicated by feeling the urge to push before full dilatation of the cervix. Pushing at this stage is detrimental to good progress in labour, especially if the fetus is presenting by the breech. Therefore any modification of breathing patterns is directed against the instinctive reaction to hold one's breath. Teaching a way to cope with this usually involves a distraction technique, such as singing a nursery rhyme or other familiar song, counting to ten repeatedly, tapping a rhythm or using a breathing pattern such as 'Hoo, Hoo, Ha, Ha'.

Relaxation and Breathing for Labour

(h) BREATHING FOR THE SECOND STAGE OF LABOUR

During the second stage the efficiency of the expulsive contractions is influenced by the mother's breathing and position (see Chapter 7). Second stage breathing and pushing has received a large amount of attention from a wide variety of groups: obstetricians, physiologists, physiotherapists, midwives, paediatricians and lay groups such as the National Childbirth Trust, and mothers themselves.

The priorities are:

A fetus who is not compromised.
A mother who is making best use of her energy resources and feels in control of herself.

Reflect on the factors that should influence what you teach. Are you familiar with the traditional exhortation to a mother 'push hard, keep it going, keep it going,' as she gets redder and redder in the face? Finally she gasps in a quick breath as she is told, 'Come along, push down again, don't waste your contraction.' This is an example of the Valsalva Manoeuvre.[17] While she holds her breath her blood pressure is lowered, there is a reduction in oxygenated blood circulating and the carbon dioxide level rises; the red face is due to venous congestion. The quick gasp of air is followed by a rebound rise in blood pressure with possible profound effects on maternal circulation. What is happening to the fetus in the meantime? The short answer is hypoxia.[18] Shorter pushes, the mother taking as many breaths as she needs, can lead to more effective, less strenuous pushing.[19]

Pushing accompanied by an outbreath is efficient.[20] Those practising yoga have long been taught to exhale before the strenuous movements in the postures. Yoga also discourages any control of breathing that causes stress.[21] Sportsmen and their coaches are also aware of the empowering capacity of the outbreath on exertion; think of karate exponents and

Relaxation and Breathing for Labour

even tennis players who serve with a grunt.

It may also be helpful for mothers to realize that contractions in the second stage may not all be of equal intensity, may peak twice during a contraction, or may be felt in surges of intensity.[22] It can be disturbing if events don't happen as they expect and they may worry unnecessarily because of variations of the normal. Second stage contractions do follow one another closely and mothers sometimes say, 'It seemed like one long contraction, no break in between.' You can teach them to use the short breaks as positive rest periods.

The light breaths requested of the mother at the time of the delivery of the head are not difficult for her to learn or remember. The image of the panting dog is one many midwives use. Many women fear perineal tears and this can inhibit pushing at this time. The sensation of a stretching perineum can be anticipated to some extent by putting a finger in each corner of the mouth and pulling hard for a few seconds.

(i)..

Can you think of anything else clients may need or want to know?

4 How Are You Going To Teach?

Before you start teaching relaxation, ask your clients to discuss briefly the reasons for tension and what it can do to the individual. By encouraging them to experience tension in the session and reflect on situations in their own lives which cause them to be tense, they can be helped to see the need for the skill you propose to teach them.

Before starting to teach breathing for labour clients could be asked to discuss their feelings and knowledge about labour. Understanding the reasons why you believe awareness and modification of breathing is useful may help to make them

Relaxation and Breathing for Labour

more receptive to your suggestions. Rehearsing breathing through a contraction sometimes produces hilarity because of the unreality of the situation. There is no reason why the classes cannot be fun, but you do want the mothers to feel there is a useful purpose behind what you ask them to do.

Consider what position the mothers are in when you teach them to relax. It is probably easiest to achieve relaxation lying down, with the body fully supported. Think of the many occasions when relaxation is needed and lying down is not possible. Relaxation can be practised in many different positions and it is useful to introduce this concept to your clients.

While complete silence is not necessary or even desirable in an environment for teaching relaxation, it is probably easier to learn in a room that is free from excessive extraneous noise and interruptions. In labour and in many

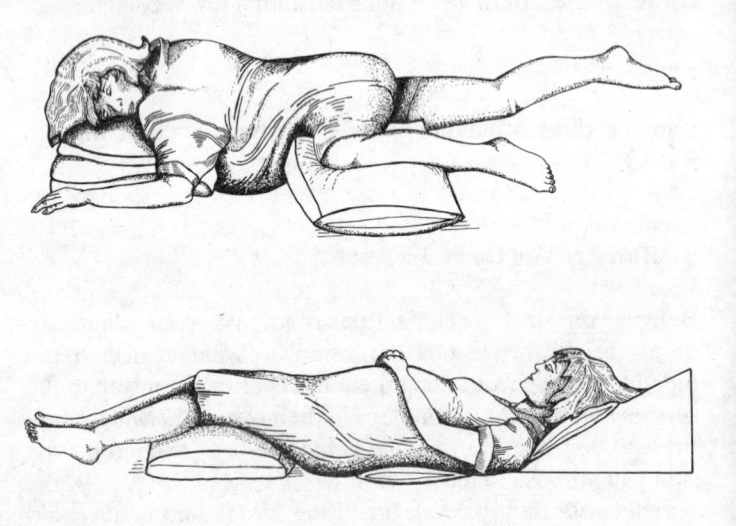

Figure 6.1 Positions for relaxing

Relaxation and Breathing for Labour

other situations relaxation may have to be practised in the presence of distractions and this can be done successfully.

Is the room warm and well ventilated? It is not easy to relax if you are cold and, once relaxed, the body will lose heat.[23] Neither is a stuffy room conducive to comfort.

Is the tone, pitch and pace of your voice appropriate? A quasi-hypnotic voice is not necessary or useful; you are giving instructions for clients to follow, not trying to mesmerize them. A calm, smooth, clear and moderately quiet delivery is probably most suitable.[24] You may find it helpful to listen to a tape recording of yourself giving the instructions.

The acquisition of a skill needs practice. You need to think about how you will encourage clients to practise. You could teach relaxation once, possibly with one revision, and then encourage them to practise alone. You could practise at several sessions or even include a short relaxation period at every session. If you do this, think whether it would be appropriate at the end of the session or at the beginning.

When you are teaching breathing rhythms or patterns try not to dictate the pace. If you are able to phrase your instructions in a way that encourages each client to follow at her own pace, it should be easier for her to learn and remember.

Think about how you will rehearse breathing through a contraction. You could ask clients to imagine a contraction, talking through a timed contraction, using visual images such as increasingly rough seas or climbing a hill that is getting steeper. You could ask them to work in pairs, taking it in turn to provide a distraction against which the other concentrates on correct breathing. A distraction could be a painful stimulus such as a pinch on the thigh for the length of a contraction. Hand pressure on either side of the lower rib cage, increasing and decreasing the pressure to simulate the pattern of intensity of the contractions is a useful way of practising breathing before labour. If Braxton Hicks'

Relaxation and Breathing for Labour

contractions become uncomfortable in later pregnancy this is a suitable time to practise breathing techniques.

Breathing for labour may be taught at one session, with revision at a later time. Since different techniques are used at different stages of labour, it may be easier for clients to learn and remember if these are taught at different times. Remember, skills need practice; allow time for repetition. Something that needs to be recalled in a time of stress should be learned so thoroughly that response is almost automatic. Groups and individuals will vary in how long they take to understand and learn a skill; build flexibility into your planning for sessions.

5 What Aids Will You Need?

Large foam wedges are useful in providing comfortable support in both lying and sitting positions.
Large bean bags are versatile. If these will be available during labour, clients can be encouraged to experiment with different positions which may be comfortable at that time.
The type of chairs you have are unlikely to be ideal, so cushions or shaped back supports are useful.
A large number of pillows is also invaluable.
If the room is not carpeted, mats will be needed.
Drawings or overhead projection transparencies depicting a contraction as a wave line, overlaid with a pattern of breathing appropriate for different stages of labour, are useful.[25]
Consider showing a video of labouring women, demonstrating breathing in labour.
Ask a recently delivered mother to talk of her own experiences and answer questions.

See list in Chapter 7 for other teaching aids for labour.

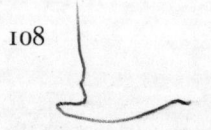

Relaxation and Breathing for Labour

6 Trigger Questions For Discussion

How would you body react if there was a loud explosion just outside the window?
What would your body feel like if you had just realized you had lost your purse?
If you can think of a time when you felt angry or frightened or in pain, do you remember what it felt like?
In what situations do you feel tense?
(Demonstrate a position of tension.) Do I look comfortable and relaxed? What tells you I am not relaxed?
(After a relaxation session.) Can you describe how you feel?
In what situations do you think you could use that technique?
Why do you think I want to teach you how to breathe in labour?
If you have seen a mother in labour on a video, what did you think of the way she was breathing?
Have friends who have had babies told you anything about breathing in labour?

7 How Will You Know When You Have Achieved Your Aims And Objectives?

You need to think about how you will know if relaxation has been achieved. If you lift a client's limb when she is relaxed, it will drop heavily when you let go. If she is not fully relaxed, she will take the weight and not allow it to drop. If you observe the women during the session, the attitude of their bodies, whether they move or are still, their facial expressions, eye movements, will all give you clues as to their state of relaxation. A discussion at the end of the session will allow clients to review how they felt and help them to be aware of when they achieve a state of relaxation and when they do not.

Clients should be able to demonstrate different patterns of

breathing appropriate to the stages of labour. You could demonstrate inappropriate breathing patterns, and then ask the women to correct your breathing. You may wish them to show confidence that breathing appropriately will help them to cope with labour. A discussion will give clients the opportunity to do this.

If you have the opportunity to be with any of your clients in labour, this will give you an excellent chance to assess their learning and evaluate your teaching. Feedback from mothers after delivery either in person or by questionnaire can provide useful information. If you are able to organize a reunion meeting after the birth, the group can report back their feelings and experiences.

References

1 Iyengar, B. K. S. (1966), *Light on Yoga*, Unwin, London, pp. 422–3; 432.
2 Hewitt, J. (1978), *Teach Yourself Meditation*, Hodder and Stoughton, Sevenoaks, pp. 60–6.
3 Madders, J. (1979), *Stress and Relaxation*, Macdonald Optima, London, pp. 48–60.
4 Ibid., pp. 70–1.
5 Williams, M. and Booth, D. (1985), *Antenatal Education. Guidelines for Teachers*, 3rd edn, Churchill Livingstone, London, pp. 97–8.
6 Madders, J. (1979), *Stress and Relaxation*, pp. 74–5.
7 Kitzinger, S. (1977), *Education and Counselling for Childbirth*, Baillière Tindall, London, pp. 156–61.
8 Mitchell, L. (1987), *Simple Relaxation. The Mitchell Method for Easing Tension*, 2nd edn, John Murray, London, pp. 42–43.
9 Ibid., pp. 60–62. (Published by permission of Laura Mitchell and John Murray (Publishers) Ltd.)
10 Ibid., cassette available from: Laura Mitchell, 8 Gainsborough Gardens, Well Walk, London NW3 1BJ. Price £5.50 including postage, packing and VAT.
11 Benson, H. (1976), *The Relaxation Response*, Collins, Glasgow, pp. 62–8.

12. Noble, E. (1982), *Essential Exercises for the Childbearing Year*, 2nd edn, John Murray, London, pp. 141–6.
13. Saling, E. and Lidgas, P. (1969), 'The effect on the fetus of maternal hyperventilation during labour', *Journal of Obstetrics and Gynaecology of the British Commonwealth*, vol. 76, October, pp. 877–80.
14. Williams, M. and Booth, D. (1985), *Antenatal Education*, 3rd edn, Churchill Livingstone, London, p. 175.
15. Noble, *Essential Exercises for the Childbearing Year*, p. 144.
16. Moir, D. M. (1982), *Pain Relief in Labour. A Handbook for Midwives*, Churchill Livingstone, Edinburgh, p. 61.
17. Inch, S. (1982), *Birthrights. A Parents' Guide to Modern Childbirth*, Hutchinson, London, p. 125.
18. Ibid., pp. 126–7.
19. Kitzinger, S. (1977), *Education and Counselling for Childbirth*, p. 191.
20. Inch, S. (1982), *Birthrights. A Parents' Guide to Modern Childbirth*, p. 128.
21. Iyengar, *Light on Yoga*, p. 59.
22. Kitzinger, *Education and Counselling for Childbirth*, p. 234.
23. Mitchell, *Simple Relaxation. The Mitchell Method for Easing Tension*, p. 44.
24. Ibid., p. 43.
25. Williams and Booth, *Antenatal Education*, pp. 135–40.

Further Reading

Balaskas, J. (1983), *Active Birth*, Unwin, London.
Dale, B. and Roeber, J. (1982), *Exercises for Childbirth*, Century, London.
Lawrence, H. (1988), 'Breathing for labour', *Journal of the Association of Chartered Physiotherapists in Obstetrics and Gynaecology*, no. 62, January, pp. 21–3.
Turton, P. (1986), 'Relaxation techniques', *Nursing*, vol. 3, no. 9, September, pp. 348–51.

7
Labour and Birth

The need to know how to cope with labour and birth is probably the main reason most women attend antenatal classes. Think how best you can serve their interests. You can prepare the mother so that she is able to take an active and informed role in her labour and prepare her companion to give emotional and psychological support. The physiological processes of labour are enhanced when the mother's anxiety is reduced and she is an active participant in her labour.[1,2] Will you prepare your clients to accept routine care? Or will you encourage them to share in the decision-making with the care givers? Consider your role if clients wish to challenge standard practices.

1 What Are Your Aims?

Clients will be able to:

Show they have the knowledge to maximize their own coping skills during labour.
Show they are prepared for the experience of labour and the procedures they may encounter.
Take part in making decisions about how their labours are conducted.
Show a positive attitude to labour and birth.
Or . . .?

Having your aims in mind,

Labour and Birth

2 What Are Your Objectives?

At the end of the session the mothers will be able to:

Recall the process of normal labour.
Discuss their hopes and fears for labour.
Demonstrate a knowledge of labour ward procedures.
Demonstrate recognition of the roles of the midwife and doctor.
Recall the available methods of pain relief in labour.
Discuss the relative merits of pain relief methods.
Or . . . ?

3 What Are You Going To Teach?

(a) SIGNS OF LABOUR AND ADMISSION TO HOSPITAL

As the beginning of labour is often an ill-defined event and may occur in a a variety of ways, it is helpful to discuss this with your clients. Think about what would be useful for the women to know. You could discuss the 'show'; they need to know its significance, what it looks like and what they should do if they observe one. While reassuring them of the normality of a small amount of blood in a 'show', you should take care not to make them so complacent that they disregard an antepartum haemorrhage. The rupturing of the membranes is also a cause for concern; women want to know when it may happen and how great a volume of fluid may be lost. Because there is no warning of this event, they worry about the embarrassment of membranes rupturing in a public place. One practical point to raise is the protection of their mattresses at home.

Concern is often shown by clients about labour starting without them being aware they are having contractions. The women may attribute backache or abdominal pain to a cause

Labour and Birth

other than labour at first. It may reassure clients to know this may happen without any ill-effects to themselves. It may also be useful to discuss the concept of 'false' or 'pre-' labour. Although contractions often start at low intensity and are widely spaced, the possibility that contractions may be strong and close together from the beginning could be mentioned. It can add to a woman's distress if she believes this is abnormal.

It is difficult to be precise about the timing of admission to hospital but it would be useful to give them guidelines to help them decide. They should be clear about those signs which may herald a potential problem, such as bleeding from the vagina, and what action they should take. Some clients worry about the possibility of precipitate labour. Questions on this should be answered, but think about whether you will raise this subject if your clients do not.

When women are in labour they need to know exactly who to contact, where in the hospital to go when they arrive and if the arrangements are different at night. If you are teaching in the community and your clients are attending more than one hospital, consider whether you will obtain that information for them or instruct them how to find out for themselves.

Ask your clients to think about how they will travel to hospital in labour. If they have a car, they will need to know what the parking arrangements are at the hospital. If they will need an ambulance, check they know how to obtain one. If they live in an area covered by a different ambulance service to the hospital, special arrangements may have to be made in advance. Some women may contemplate driving themselves to hospital in labour. You could raise this point in order to dissuade them, because there is potential risk to them and their baby if labour suddenly escalates or something untoward happens.

Much of this may seem common sense but every woman may not know what seems obvious to you. For example, every woman may not realize she can telephone and talk to a

Labour and Birth

midwife at any time of the day or night. Clear information about such simple practical matters will hopefully help to make the onset of labour relatively panic-free.

(b) PHYSIOLOGY OF LABOUR

Some understanding of what is happening to their bodies should help clients cope with the stress of labour – most of us fear the unknown. But you need to think about how much they want or need to know. Groups will vary in the amount of information they require and it may not be obvious at first; well-educated women may not want as much detail as they are capable of learning and less well-educated women can ask some very searching questions. You need to assess each group rather than make assumptions.

Think of the words you use: womb or uterus, neck of the womb or cervix, afterbirth or placenta, delivery or birth. Maybe both, so they understand what they may hear said when they are in labour. Even if they fully understand the medical term, you may consider the word in common use to be more appropriate.

The length of labour is something most women want to know about. Impossible to forecast, but it is not helpful to be unrealistic. When discussing the length of labour it is well to consider the different interpretations that can be made about the start of labour. Imagine a woman coming into hospital having had contractions for several hours, intermittently at first then regular. On examination her midwife judges she is not yet established in labour. The contractions continue intermittently, finally becoming established and labour is completed over twenty-four hours after admission. The mother may interpret this as a labour lasting nearly two days, whereas the midwife records a labour of seventeen hours.

It is almost impossible to convey to another woman what labour feels like, even when you have experienced labour yourself. The backache or period-like pains of early labour is

Labour and Birth

easy enough to understand but the overwhelming nature of the later contractions is more difficult. Visual images such as 'riding a wave' or 'climbing a mountain' can help.[3] Few women can reach labour without some idea of contractions or 'labour pains', but some may have only a very hazy notion of the purpose of those contractions and how they are dilating the cervix.

Think about what you have observed of the physical and emotional state of women in transition. Think whether you will warn them of the possibility of shaking, vomiting, irrational behaviour, the feeling of not being able to go on or wanting to push before the cervix is fully dilated.

The sensations of the contractions of the second stage are described as pushing or bearing down. 'Like having your bowels open' is another description, but mothers are often unprepared for feeling that is exactly what they do want to do. This can inhibit their pushing effort and cause great distress about 'making a mess'. Teaching a woman to be aware of what her body is doing, helping her to have confidence in her body's capabilities, will lead to better teamwork between mother and midwife, so enhancing the birth experience.[4] Many women know that an epidural can obliterate the desire to push, but do not realize the absence of a desire to push may happen naturally.

If a mother wishes to try squatting during the second stage, ask if she is supple enough to squat comfortably. Most western women gave up squatting by the time they were five years old, and will need to practise before it is once again an easy and comfortable position. Physiological considerations point to an upright position being the one of choice in the second stage; gravity aids descent of the presenting part and there is increased efficiency of uterine contractions.[5] Squatting increases the size of pelvic outlet.[6] Interference in maternal circulation with consequent compromise of the fetus can occur in a supine position[7] and there is a risk of low back strain in the lithotomy position.[8] Understanding these factors

Labour and Birth

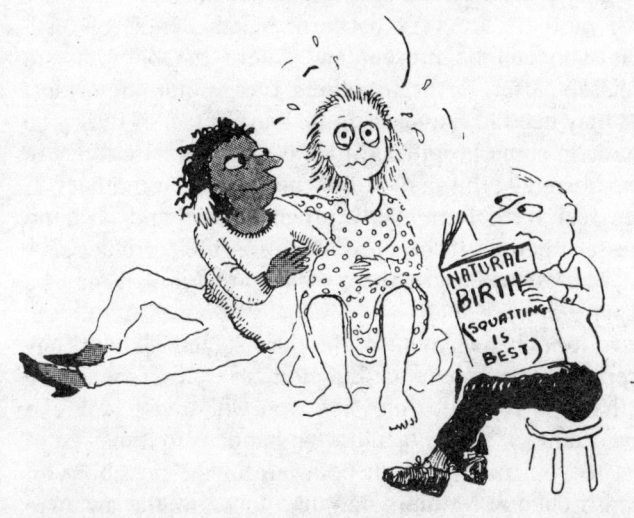

can help mothers to think for themselves and also to be responsive to a midwife's guidance. Changing position in labour can seem a terrible effort, but if the woman is able to recollect or can be reminded of the reason, she may be more willing to try.

Midwives differ in the way they encourage the mothers to push. Maybe with lungs full, closed glottis and lots of encouragement for long hard pushes, or maybe they encourage shorter pushes with several quick breaths in between, being less directive and expecting the mother to respond to her own body. It can be confusing if a mother has been taught one method antenatally and then finds herself being encouraged to do something different (see Chapter 6).

Think about how much clients want to know about how a baby is born. They may want to know less detail of how a baby moves through the pelvis and more about how they will feel as it happens, or what the midwife will expect them to

Labour and Birth

do. Your beautiful explanation of the mechanism of birth will fall on deaf ears if all they are thinking is, 'I'm so scared that I shall rip in half when the baby comes through.'

Some mothers are very concerned with details of birth such as who will be present and where the baby is laid immediately after birth; to others this is not important. Clients may need to request skin-to-skin contact or it may be automatic in some hospitals. Student observers are likely in training hospitals; this may or may not matter to mothers. If couples feel birth is a highly private event and wish no unnecessary people to be present, this is their privilege. A special request to ensure their wishes are fulfilled may be necessary.

The routine management of the third stage of labour may be acceptable to your clients. If a mother requests something other than the routine, think how you will advise her. The appearance of the placenta and what happens to it may be of interest to your mothers, but be aware of the possibility of squeamish clients. Mothers may like to know the arrangements after the birth for rest and refreshment, time alone with their partner and transfer to the postnatal ward.

(c) COPING STRATEGIES

Consider what attitudes to pain in labour you will try to foster: 'I can and will manage without any drugs.' 'I will accept pain relief from the staff as soon as I feel I need it.' 'I will accept pain relief from the staff only if I am really desperate.' 'I will wait and see what happens and then make up my mind.' Most women expect some degree of pain in labour and it would be unrealistic of antenatal teachers to deny this happens to the majority of women in the 'civilized' world. It would also be unrealistic to teach the mothers to believe that antenatal preparation and self-help techniques will ensure a pain-free labour. If the expectation of a pain-free labour without drugs is not fulfilled, a mother can feel

Labour and Birth

cheated and angry. However, with preparation women can help themselves to minimize the pain and make maximum use of all available coping strategies. It is useful to introduce to them the concept of being aware of, and in tune with, their bodies. This will allow them to go along with labour, instead of fighting it.

Position, or rather positions, since no one position will be comfortable for the whole of labour, are important. Few would argue that good positioning cannot contribute to a woman's comfort in labour and, as mentioned, there is evidence that an upright position can have an advantageous effect on the efficiency of uterine contractions. Trials have not proved conclusively whether ambulation is cause or

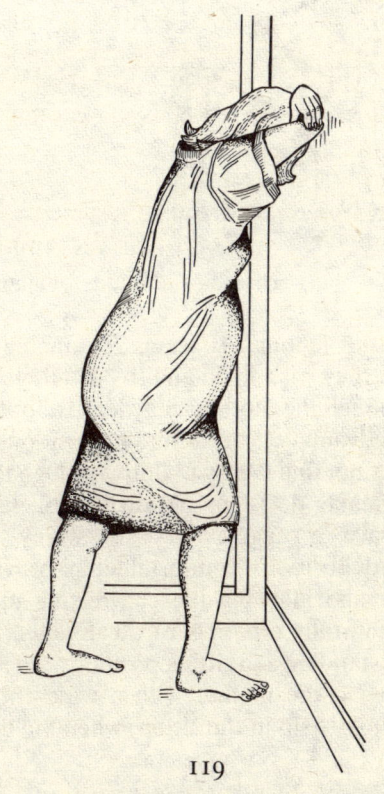

Labour and Birth

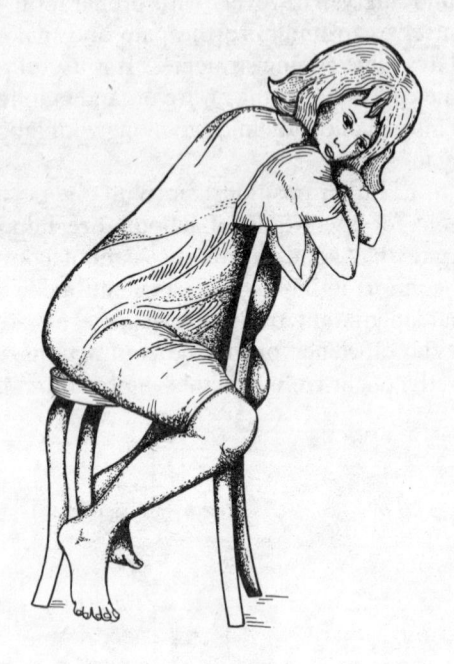

Fig. 7.1 Forward leaning positions for labour

effect of an easier labour.[9] It seems reasonable to support women in what they wish to do and to encourage them to be active. Even though the mothers may learn about the advantages and disadvantages of different positions, when in labour they may not find it easy to think through the situation logically and make decisions. Midwives or labour companions may have to suggest and assist. Many women find leaning forward positions comfortable in providing relief from backache and allowing the contracting uterus to tip forward as it naturally attempts to do. Leaning forward in many different standing and sitting positions can be practised in class to provide the mother with a wide choice.[10] One position which may help in transition, when the urge to push

Labour and Birth

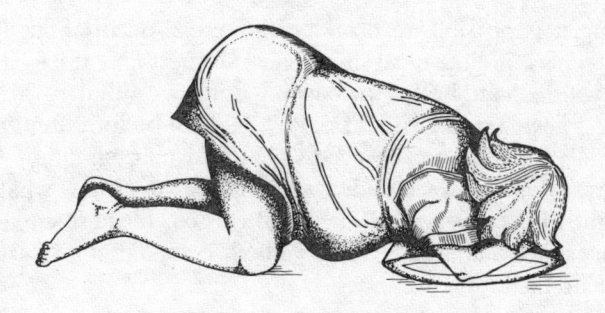

Fig. 7.2 Helpful position to relieve back when the urge to push comes before full dilatation

is felt before full dilatation of the cervix, is kneeling with the head on the same level as the knees and the pelvis raised.[11]

Many of the advantages of good positioning apply also to movement. While few women will walk around for the whole of labour, many will find movement helpful in the early stages, and this includes pelvic rocking and rotation.[12] Before you encourage your clients to make plans to stay mobile through labour you should warn them of possible restrictions: not only the obvious ones of fetal monitoring and syntocinon infusion, but also any particular restrictions of individual hospitals or individuals within them.

Relaxation will not only help them to cope with the pain of labour, it will help to promote a better use of their resources, which can influence the outcome of labour. Every midwife must have seen the mother who is too exhausted to push her baby out without the use of forceps. Better conservation of her energy earlier in labour might have enabled her to deliver normally (see Chapter 6). Lying in a bath of warm water can be soothing and relaxing.[13]

Breathing rhythms for labour should be simple and thoroughly learnt if they are to be effective. It is also necessary for those assisting the mother in labour to know what breathing techniques she has been taught (see Chapter 6).

Labour and Birth

While it is possible to do a 'crash course' once labour has started, it is not the ideal situation.[14] Mothers may still forget, but will respond better to coaching if it is a reminder, rather than a new learning situation. It should not be forgotten that the labour ward is, of necessity, a learning situation for many.[15] Labour ward midwives do not always know what is taught to the mothers in antenatal classes. In these circumstances the role of an informed labour companion is of great value to the mother.

Massage is a widely used method of comfort and pain relief in many situations.[16] Deep back massage is often effective when the pain of labour is predominantly in the back. Effleurage on the abdomen can be soothing, but women in labour differ in their desire for physical contact. Some may not want to be touched by either midwife or labour companion. It can be helpful to encourage the idea that it is acceptable for them to state their likes and dislikes when they are in labour.

(d) PAIN RELIEF

Pharmacological pain relief is freely available, but women are concerned about its effect on themselves and their babies. Be prepared to discuss all the advantages and disadvantages of different methods.[17,18] If you acknowledge that the responsibility for making decisions about pain relief lies in part with the mother, you need to give her all the facts if she is to make an informed choice. Consider how you will resolve any conflict between what you believe about the use of pain-relieving drugs and the official policies of your clients' hospitals.

Pethidine is an option in most hospitals, given in standard doses. A woman may wish to know if she may request a smaller-than-usual dose. The policy regarding the administration of pethidine at different degrees of cervical dilatation is also important. Details of other drugs such as tranquillizers or anti-emetics which are likely to be offered also need consideration.

Labour and Birth

Transcutaneous electrical nerve stimulation (TENS) activates the body's own pain-relieving capacity as endorphin and encephalin are produced. It also works by using the 'gate theory' of pain control.[19] It has been used for many years to help those suffering pain through a variety of medical conditions, but is not yet available in every maternity unit. Some obstetricians, midwives and, particularly, obstetric physiotherapists[20] are familiar with its use. The electrodes through which the pulse is administered are placed on the woman's back at the levels of the roots of the sensory nerve supply of

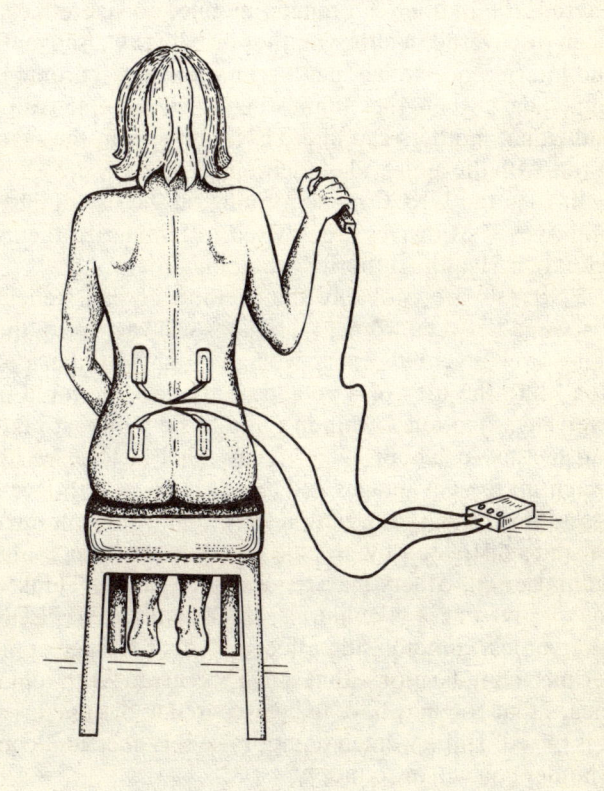

Fig. 7.3 TENS in use

Labour and Birth

the uterus and the cervix. There is a range of frequencies and rates at which the pulse can be administered, which can be controlled by the mother. Most women who try TENS find it gives some relief; for some it will be adequate for the whole of labour, for others it gives relief for only part of the time. Some obtain little or no relief and a few women dislike the sensation.

Many studies in various parts of the world have evaluated the use of TENS.[21] The advantages of TENS are: no restrictions on the length of time it can be used, no drug is administered, the mother can remain mobile, no side-effects have been discovered in either mother or baby. A disadvantage is the interference which may occur with the recording of the fetal heart when the monitoring is via a fetal scalp clip. Individual mothers can hire TENS units from the manufacturers with the approval of their obstetrician.

In 1986 the UKCC made a ruling on the use of TENS by midwives.[22] Midwives are advised to familiarize themselves with their Health Authority's standing orders.

Epidurals are probably the method of pain relief most discussed between women. Opinions will vary from 'the best thing ever invented, every woman's right' to 'dangerous, I don't like the idea of a needle in my back, I would never, ever have one' or 'I wouldn't like to be numb, it takes the satisfaction of labour away'. They need facts to be able to weigh up the advantages and disadvantages, but once again assess how much information they want. Some women can be quite distressed by graphic details of how an epidural is administered, others may request such detail. Think about the disadvantages of epidurals; it is reasonable to discuss the more or less common side-effects. Media coverage of the few serious complications that have occurred with epidurals means that you may have to be prepared to discuss this also if it is raised. If the women do not raise this question, consider whether you will introduce it.

A client may be adamant about not having an epidural in

Labour and Birth

labour. You may feel it is worth encouraging her not to close her mind completely to the possibility. You and she cannot know in advance what type of labour she will experience. If, after being determined to have a drug-free labour, she finally accepts an epidural or other pain relief, disappointment and a sense of failure may ensue. Some teachers, however, believe that by introducing the idea that she may not be able to cope, you diminish her chances of doing so.

The Entonox mixture of 50 per cent nitrous oxide and 50 per cent oxygen is still referred to sometimes as 'gas and air'. It is useful for women to realize the significance of the difference in the percentage of oxygen they receive between gas and air, and gas and oxygen; also, that it may be administered by mask or mouthpiece. Although the practice of restricting the length of time Entonox is used in labour does not appear to be well founded,[23] this may happen in some hospitals.

Other methods of pain relief such as acupuncture, hypnosis or homoeopathy are sometimes used. These methods may be acceptable to the obstetricians and midwives if they are forewarned, and the mother provides her own practitioner.

(e) LABOUR WARD PROCEDURES AND POLICIES

If a mother wishes to challenge the standard practice, think about how you will help her. Should you encourage her, and give her all the available information to enable her to state her case fully, or should you persuade her to accept what is the norm for that hospital? Health educators should not be the 'yes men/women' of the medical establishment. They have a duty to seek to change what they believe is wrong. Consumer demand can work effectively to bring about change, but the labour ward should not be a battleground.

An experienced midwife will have developed her own professional opinions about various policies and practices in midwifery. She may find herself at odds with other midwives

Labour and Birth

or obstetricians. How far, as an antenatal teacher, can she go in putting forward her own ideas, where they clash with what the clients will encounter? However well-founded her opinions, if her teaching results in a lack of trust by the clients in those caring for them, the outcome may be an unhappy experience. Carers are unlikely to give of their best in an atmosphere of antagonism. Health educators in the USA felt that, 'producing dissonance between people and the society in which they must function is usually neither useful or kind'.[24] Nevertheless a woman who makes requests, either of her own volition, or as a result of your teaching, can be helped to fulfil them. You can help her to formulate her requests in a lucid and assertive but non-aggressive manner,[25] and get to know the best people for her to approach, well before labour. A labouring woman is not at her best for conducting negotiations. Since, however, even with the most willing of midwives and obstetricians, labour plans may be upset by problems, women should be helped to accept such deviation without too much disappointment.

Procedures which are part of a midwife's daily routine can be worrying to mothers if they do not understand them and the reasons for them. Articulate women may have no problem in asking for explanations, but others may accept such procedures without question, in spite of anxiety. Acquiring knowledge of routine procedures is only part of the answer; as important is acquiring the confidence to ask questions.

Queries are often raised by clients about perineal shaving and enemas. It would be helpful if you were familiar with the policies in the hospitals your clients attend.

Eating and drinking in labour is another concern. The common hospital practice of withholding all food and fluids, except small amounts of water, from labouring women has become so well known that some women will starve themselves at home even before labour is established. Certainly large or rich meals during early labour may lead to vomiting later. But a diet of small amounts of mainly carbohydrate

Labour and Birth

foods, low in fibre and free from fat, with fluids as desired, is probably the best advice for early labour, according to present knowledge. The risk of pulmonary aspiration is a danger in general anaesthesia.[26] The effects of starvation in labour can be a problem. The need to be prepared for an emergency general anaesthetic, used as a justification for the practice of severely restricting oral alimentation in all labouring women, is still a matter for debate.[27,28,29] It will be helpful if the mother is aware of the policy of the hospital where she will give birth.

The amount of fetal monitoring carried out in normal labours varies considerably. Different criteria influence the decision to monitor the fetal heart externally or internally. Different methods of monitoring contractions can be used. Fetal scalp blood sampling may be done. Mothers react differently to being monitored electronically. This will depend on personal philosophy on interventions, knowledge of its purpose and how monitoring is handled by the staff who are caring for them. The equipment can restrict movement, but this can be circumvented if radio telemetry is available. Mothers may be helped if you are able to familiarize them with the appearance and sound of the machinery. The sound of their baby's heart beat can be reassuring to some mothers, but not all. Can you with certainty answer the question, 'Does it hurt the baby when a fetal scalp electrode is put on?' You may like to consider trying to put one on your own scalp. Mothers may also wish to know if the electrode will mark the baby's head.

Policies vary on the frequency of vaginal examinations, and when they will be done by a midwife and when by a doctor. Artificial rupture of membranes is sometimes done routinely or alternatively at the discretion of the midwife or doctor. It would be useful for the mother to know if her permission for this procedure is actively sought, or her tacit consent assumed. You could discuss the relative merits of labouring with intact or ruptured membranes. It is important for clients to be aware of the factors which can be influenced by the condition of the membranes, such as length of labour, severity of the pain of contractions, formation of caput succedaneum, moulding and fetal monitoring.[30]

Episiotomy and the circumstances under which it will be performed is of great concern to many mothers. One study has suggested that perineal massage can reduce the need for episiotomy.[31] This may be a technique for your clients to consider.

One option which mothers may wish to think about is 'Leboyer birth'. Provision may be made to accommodate mothers who wish for some or all aspects of Leboyer's ideas of how birth should be conducted. Different types of bed, chair or stool may be available for the birth. It will be helpful if mothers are aware of what restrictions, if any, will be placed on the positions they may wish to adopt for labour and birth. A midwife may be happy for a mother to squat for most of the second stage, but prefer her to return to a position in which she can observe the perineum during the delivery of the head. Some women do express a desire to know more about the options available for birth position.[32]

Partners or other labour companions will be helped if they are aware of the staff's attitudes to their presence. Most hospitals will welcome or at least tolerate them. There may be some circumstances under which they may be requested to temporarily leave the labour room. It will help to make such separations more bearable if both the mother and her companion are prepared for and understand the reasons for these requests. Some hospitals may put a limit on the number of companions that may be present at any one time in the labour room (see Chapter 4).

Knowing the midwife who will deliver her, prior to labour, is not possible for many women. On a visit to the labour ward, it may be possible for your clients to meet some of the midwives who may be on duty when she delivers. If the mother sees a familiar face when she arrives on the labour

Labour and Birth

ward, this can have a beneficial effect on her state of mind. It may be helpful for her to know that she will be cared for by one or two midwives during labour, rather than a succession of different people. Do your clients know what a midwife is? This is not such a silly question as you might imagine. The duties and responsibilities of a midwife are not understood by everyone and can be equated with the role of a nurse.

If the hospital operates a birth plan scheme, your clients may wish to discuss how this should be completed.[33] Birth plans can vary from those which are non-directive, giving a few guidelines as to the type of requests a mother or couple may like to make, to others which lay down more precisely the options that are available. Mothers may or may not have the opportunity to discuss these plans with their midwives in the antenatal clinic. Birth plans could be discussed in class, even if the hospital does not print one. You could introduce the idea of writing their own. A birth plan can help clients to formulate and clarify in their own minds their hopes, fears and desires for labour.

A mother may embark upon labour with the highest expectations of a joyful, satisfying experience, determined to cope using only her own resources. If she then has a long, painful labour needing pain relief, consider how she may feel. She may feel very unhappy, reluctant to accept the situation, perhaps frustrated, disappointed and have a sense of failure. It is not helpful to prepare a mother to expect agonizing pain and reliance on drugs. But you should encourage the woman to have a positive attitude, with realistic expectations and an open mind. You could explore some of the reasons why a labour may be prolonged or painful – for example, if the fetus is in the occipito-posterior position.

(f) MEDICAL INTERVENTION

Mothers may ask if they will be attended by doctors they know or by whichever doctor or team is on call for that day,

Labour and Birth

or whether a female doctor will be available.

It can be difficult to strike the right note when introducing what happens when all is not normal and straightforward. In a group you may have a 'worrier' who is anxious, asks many questions about possible problems, but seems to gain little reassurance from increased knowledge. Others may gain confidence from knowing what the likely deviations from the normal are and about their management. Or a denial mechanism may operate and prevent assimilation of the information presented. Those who have a particular problem may just want to know what will be done for that and have little interest in any other abnormalities.

The criteria used to decide on induction of labour will vary, as will the methods used to induce labour. There is evidence that nipple stimulation can ripen an unfavourable cervix and accelerate a slow labour.[34] You may wish to tell your clients about this. Some hospitals will have a definite policy of active management of labour, others will tailor acceleration of labour on a more individual basis. Such policies should not come as a surprise to a woman in labour. You could discuss the fairly common problems of hypertension, ketosis and inability to pass urine and how they will be managed.

When you discuss abnormal deliveries, clients may require different amounts of detailed information, but many will want some information about what can be done to help if mother or baby face a problem. They may wish to know how a forceps delivery or ventouse extraction is carried out. This includes details such as anaesthetic options and what position they are expected to adopt. The presence of partners at abnormal deliveries could also be discussed. The differences in the management of labour if it is a twin pregnancy or if labour is pre-term could also be mentioned. A mother whose baby is presenting by the breech may wish to know the options open to her. While reassuring her that many babies will eventually turn, it may be helpful for her to know the

Labour and Birth

criteria the hospital will use to decide if a vaginal delivery will be attempted or an elective Caesarean section performed. If delivering vaginally, consider how her labour may differ from one where the baby is presenting by the vertex. For example, electronic fetal monitoring may be mandatory. Epidural analgesia is likely to be suggested to the mother as the analgesia of choice.

Consider what you will tell them about a Caesarean section: reasons why it might be performed, whether a choice of anaesthetic is available, what it feels like having a Caesarean under an epidural, and the relative merits of undergoing a Caesarean under epidural or general anaethesia. If the operation is to be performed under general anaesthesia, they may be taken into the theatre awake or asleep. Think about whether you will mention details such as catheterization, the administration of antacids and the setting up of intravenous infusions. The presence of partners and what happens to the baby after it has been born is also of concern to the mothers.

It can be helpful to describe what may be done to help a baby who does not breathe immediately. A paediatrician may carry out resuscitation where the mother or both parents can see what is happening.

Think about whether you will tell them what should be done if the labour is precipitate and the baby is born before arrival at hospital. You may feel that because it is a rare event, to discuss it would provoke unnecessary anxiety. If, however, a client is sufficiently concerned to ask, a simple, brief protocol could be suggested, with a reassurance that a quick labour is likely to be normal.

Time may restrict the amount of information you can present. Think not of your priorities, but of those of each group you teach. The amount of information available may seem overwhelming and some mothers may respond to an approach which seeks to explore their felt needs and build up their confidence rather than increasing their knowledge.

Labour and Birth

(g) ....

Can you think of anything else a client may want or need to know?

4 How Will You Teach?

An initial question and answer session can assess clients' previous knowledge and also their attitudes. You will then be able to decide on the amount of information your mothers need. When asked for immediate thoughts on labour the most common responses from women are: pain, fear, hard work, apprehension, 'I prefer not to think about it', and, sometimes, excitement and anticipation. Being given information is sometimes less important for their state of mind than sharing feelings with other mothers. It can be comforting to know you are not the only one who has what you thought was a stupid fear. Try to allow enough time for talk; it is not wasted time.

Demonstration of cervical dilatation and birth of a baby can be achieved with suitable aids.

Role play may be used to help them explore possible feelings and reactions in labour (see page 33).

If a visit to the labour ward is possible, seeing the labour ward and experiencing the atmosphere and possibly meeting some of the staff often allays some of the mother's fears. If you are teaching in the community and your clients are attending one hospital, it may be possible for you to arrange a visit as a group. If clients are attending different hospitals, you could tell them what the arrangements are for individual visits to the labour ward, or advise them how to find out.

Special considerations may apply where a straightforward labour is not anticipated, for example, with mothers expecting an elective Caesarean section or the management of labour in the presence of complications such as cardiac

Labour and Birth

disease or diabetes. You may be able to help these mothers adequately in the session, but if their particular needs are impinging on the needs of the group as a whole, you may have to consider alternatives. A short one-to-one session may enable you to meet an individual's needs. If, however, your general advice is inadequate, then the mother should be encouraged to talk directly with her obstetrician. If communication between herself and her doctor is poor, it may be necessary for you to attempt to obtain specific information about her situation.

Mothers who have suffered an interuterine death may feel unable to cope with a group, but they still have to cope with labour and may need emotional support and counselling in a one-to-one session.

Labour can cover a large amount of material; you may need more than one session to cover it adequately. You may be the sole teacher for your group or you may be working in conjunction with others, for example an obstetric physiotherapist or hospital or community midwife. If this is so, it is most helpful to the clients if you are all giving the same message. Clients will not benefit if they receive conflicting advice or perceive professionals to be at odds with one another. The Royal College of Midwives, the Health Visitors Association and the Chartered Society of Physiotherapy issued a joint statement in 1986 putting forward their desire and intention to liaise to promote the best antenatal preparation such a team approach can provide for our clients.[35]

5 What Aids Can You Use?

The number of pictorial aids, photographs, drawings, leaflets and slides available from commercial and other sources is legion (see Chapter 3 and Appendix 1). Look at them carefully and try to assess how they will be viewed by the lay person. Midwives are familiar with anatomical drawings and

Labour and Birth

diagrams. Sagittal section drawings of a fetus in the pelvis at various stages of labour may be beautifully clear to us, but think whether your clients are able to relate them to their own bodies.

Three-dimensional aids may more easily convey the information. Dilatation of the cervix is probably most easily portrayed with an aid such as a knitted uterus (see page 44). A pelvis and doll is frequently used to demonstrate birth. A miniature version is now available which is easier to manipulate single-handed, although there would be some difficulty if it was being viewed by a large group (see page 189). A pelvic floor constructed from foam plastic together with a doll can be used to show how a baby passes through (see page 46).

Think in what ways you could use your body or encourage them to use their own bodies.[36] Pulling on a polo-necked sweater or pulling a sweater sleeve over a clenched fist can be used to demonstrate cervical dilatation. You could demonstrate fetal positions. Clenched fists placed on top of one another can be used to show vertebrae and how they are positioned to aid insertion of an epidural cannula.

A visit to the labour ward may provide opportunities to demonstrate fetal monitoring equipment, use of special beds, and various other pieces of equipment that may be used.

It may be appropriate to show some or all of the following: an epidural catheter, fetal monitoring electrodes, a fetal scalp clip and an amnihook. It may be helpful if you can obtain a normal fetal monitor trace to show them.

Mothers describing their experiences, whether they are specially invited or members of the group, can be useful. But multiparae may not always wish to discuss their previous labours, so be sensitive if they show reluctance.

A video or film can provide information, promote understanding and trigger discussion. Both may give a wider variety of experience or greater realism. View what you propose to use, make your own evaluation of its usefulness, and when you show it note the reactions of the clients.[37] You

Labour and Birth

as a midwife may think a particular video gives a beautiful portrayal of labour, but it may cause distress to clients. Be prepared for clients or partners who say they do not wish to watch any films or videos; sometimes too much realism is not acceptable. Good black-and-white photographs can sometimes convey realism in a less scary way.[38]

A leaflet listing 'things to bring to hospital' may not strictly be a teaching aid but is appreciated by many mothers.

6 Trigger Questions For Discussion

What is your first thought if someone says 'labour'?
Is there one particular thing you want to know about labour?
Is there one particular thing about labour or birth that worries you?
How will you know when labour has started?
How long do you expect labour to last?
Do you expect pain in labour?
Why do you think it happens?
What can you do to help yourself cope with labour?
Have friends told you what helped them in labour?
What do you feel about having your partner with you in labour?
How does your partner feel about being with you in labour?
How would you react if, when you were constipated, you were asked to attempt opening your bowels lying on your back with your legs in the air?

To a Multipara:

Can you describe to the others what labour felt like?

7 How Will You Know When You Have Achieved Your Aims and Objectives?

If you have an objective which requires clients to discuss their hopes and fears about labour, they will have fulfilled your objective if they have the discussion; you will also be able to make a judgement about the quality of the discussion. A questionnaire on facts pertaining to labour can give you feedback about the amount of knowledge they have retained. A questionnaire or interview given soon after delivery will help you assess how useful the knowledge they gained was to them. A reunion class for the group a few weeks after delivery, in which they can look at their experiences, can give you further information about how they coped with labour.

Leaflets

A Guide to Labour for Expectant Parents, National Childbirth Trust.
The Birth, Association of Chartered Physiotherapists in Obstetrics and Gynaecology/Milupa.

References

1. Iveson-Iveson, J. (1982), 'Focus on the family, Dr Caldeyro-Barcia's childbirth methods', *Nursing Mirror*, vol. 155, no. 6, 11 August, pp. 34–6.
2. Lederman, R. P., Lederman, E., Work, B. A. and McCann, D. S. (1978), 'The relationship of maternal anxiety, plasma catecholamines, and plasma cortisol to progress in labor', *American Journal of Obstetrics and Gynecology*, vol. 132, no. 5, 1 November, pp. 495–500.
3. Kitzinger, S. (1977), *Education and Counselling for Childbirth*, Baillière Tindall, London, Frontispiece.
4. Kahana, H. (1987), *Antenatal Preparation for the Second Stage of*

Labour, International Confederation of Midwives Conference, Amsterdam, August.

5 Méndez-Bauer, C., Arroyo, J., García Ramos, C. Menéndez, A., Lavilla, M., Izquierdo, F., Villa Elízaga, I. and Zamarriego, J. (1975), 'Effects of standing position on spontaneous uterine contractility and other aspects of labor', *Journal of Perinatal Medicine*, vol. 3, pp. 89–99.

6 Russell, J. G. B. (1969), 'Moulding of the pelvic outlet', *Journal of Obstetrics and Gynaecology of the British Commonwealth*, vol. 76, pp. 817–20.

7 Johnstone, F. D., Aboelmagd, M. S. and Harouny, A. K. (1987), 'Maternal posture in the second stage and fetal acid base status', *British Journal of Obstetrics and Gynaecology,* vol. 94, pp. 753–7.

8 Inch, S. (1982), *Birthrights. A Parents' Guide to Modern Childbirth*, Hutchinson, London, pp. 121–3.

9 Inch, S. (1985), Upright posture in labour – a new orthodoxy?' *Journal of the Royal Society of Medicine*, vol. 78, no. 2, pp. 163–6.

10 Dale, B. and Roeber, J. (1982), *Exercises for Childbirth,* Century, London, pp. 98–101.

11 Ibid., p. 97.

12 Ibid., pp. 16–18.

13 Milner, I. (1988), 'Water baths for pain relief in labour', *Nursing Times,* vol. 84, no. 1, pp. 39–40.

14 Gillett, J. R. (1977), 'Helping those who have not been to preparation for childbirth classes', *Midwives Chronicle*, vol. 90, no. 1069, February, pp. 32–4.

15 Perkins, E. R. (1980), *Education for Childbirth and Parenthood*, Croom Helm, London, pp. 20–44.

16 Dale and Roeber, *Exercises for Childbirth,* pp.83–91.

17 Inch, *Birthrights. A Parents' Guide to Modern Childbirth,* pp. 100–116.

18 Moir, D. D. (1982), *Pain Relief in Labour*, Churchill Livingstone, London, pp. 19–117.

19 Melzack, R. and Wall, P. D. (1965), 'Pain mechanisms. A new theory', *Science,* vol. 150, no. 3699, pp. 971–9.

20 Polden, M. (1985), 'Transcutaneous nerve stimulation in labour and post caesarian section', *Physiotherapy*, vol. 71, no. 8, August, pp. 350–3.

21 MIDIRS (1986), *Labour and Delivery/Interventions – Pain Relief (TENS)*, December, no. 3.

22 (1986), 'UKCC Midwifery Committee Recommendation on Transcutaneous Nerve Stimulation for the relief of pain in labour', *Midwives Chronicle*, vol. 99, no. 1183, August, p. 181.

23 Inch, *Birthrights. A Parents' Guide to Modern Childbirth*, p. 107.

24 The National Center for Health Education, USA (1979), 10th International Conference on Health Education. London, HEC and King's

Fund, p. 112.
25 Dickson, A. (1982), *A Woman in Your Own Right. Assertiveness and You*, Quartet, London.
26 Douglas, M. J. (1988), 'The case against a more liberal food and fluid policy in labour', *Birth*, vol. 15, no. 2, pp. 93–4.
27 Ludka, L. (1987), *Fasting During Labour*, 21st International Confederation of Midwives Congress, August, The Hague.
28 Broach, J. and Newton, N. (1988), 'Food and beverages in labor', *Birth*, vol. 15, no. 2, June, pp. 89–92.
29 Inch, *Birthrights. A Parents' Guide to Modern Childbirth*, pp. 52–4.
30 Ibid., pp. 83–4.
31 Avery, M. and Van Arsdale, L. (1987), 'Perineal massage', *Journal of Nurse-Midwifery*, vol. 32, no. 3, May–June, pp. 181–4.
32 Gupta, J. K. and Lilford, R. J. (1987), 'Birth positions', *Midwifery*, vol. 3, no. 2, June, pp. 92–6.
33 MIDIRS (1986), *Labour and Delivery/Active Birth – Birth Plans*, July, no. 2.
34 MIDIRS (1986), *Labour and Delivery/Interventions – Breast Stimulation*, March, no. 1; December, no. 3.
35 RCM, HVA, CSP (1987), 'Working together in psychophysical preparation for childbirth', *The Association of Chartered Physiotherapists in Obstetrics and Gynaecology Journal*, no. 61, July, p. 4.
36 Deane Gray, T. (1986), 'The application of audio visual aids in everyday parenthood education', *Maternal and Child Health*, vol. 11, no. 10, pp. 342–4.
37 Archer, R. (1988), 'Why I Dislike Birth Films', *International Journal of Childbirth Education*, vol. 2, no. 3, May, pp. 31–2.
38 Durrell McKenna, N. (1988), *Birth. A Unique Visual Record–14 Different Births in Hospital, at Home, Caesarian, Epidural, Breech, Twins*, Bloomsbury, London.

Further Reading

Balaskas, J. (1983), *Active Birth*, Unwin, London.
Kitzinger, S. (1987), *Freedom and Choice in Childbirth*, Viking/Penguin, Harmondsworth.
Melzack, R. (1973), *The Puzzle of Pain*, Penguin, Harmondsworth.
Melzack, R. and Wall, P. D. (1982), *The Challenge of Pain*, Penguin, Harmondsworth.
Milner, I. (1986), 'Choosing a natural or an active childbirth', *Nursing*, vol. 3, no. 2, February, pp. 39–45.

Riley, E. M. D. (1977), 'What do women want? – the question of choice in the conduct of labour'. In: *Benefits and Hazards of the New Obstetrics*, Chard, T. and Richards, M. (eds), Heinemann, London, pp. 62–71.

Thomson, A. M. (1988), 'Management of the woman in normal second stage of labour: a review', *Midwifery*, vol. 4, pp. 77–85.

8
Baby Care and Feeding

A baby's basic needs – food, love, warmth and hygiene – will be supplied by its mother. Midwives and doctors are there to complement and supplement the care but the mother is the prime carer. Mothers today often are not able to learn basic baby care skills by observation and participation in the life of an extended family. Think how you can help to foster mothers' confidence and assist them to start learning the skills of baby care. It is well to bear in mind that practical skills are best learnt by practice and it is difficult for a mother to be able to do this before her baby is born. An understanding of the basic psychology of the newborn may help a mother to interact more fully with her baby.

1 What Are Your Aims?

Clients will be able to:

Make an informed decision about the method of feeding their babies.
Care adequately for their babies.
Show a confident attitude to their forthcoming role as parents.
Or . . . ?

Having your aims in mind,

Baby Care and Feeding

2 What Are Your Objectives?

At the end of the session the mother will be able to:

List the advantages and disadvantages of breast- and bottle-feeding.
Identify possible problems in the early weeks of feeding.
Recall the factors that aid successful breastfeeding.
Demonstrate confidence in her ability to care for her baby.
Discuss a baby's basic needs.
Recognize possible minor health problems of the early weeks.
Recall a newborn baby's capabilities.
Recall how a baby becomes attached to his or her mother.
Or . . . ?

3 What Will You Teach?

(a) CHOICE OF FEEDING METHOD

When discussing choice of feeding method, think whether you as a teacher will try to be impartial, giving an unbiased view. Or, alternatively, state any bias you may have, acknowledging the equal validity of both their opinions and your own. Some antenatal teachers believe it is not helpful to ask women to state their intention at this time, feeling that it puts unwarranted pressure on decision-making.

The choice of feeding method will be influenced by cultural background, family and peer-group influences and personal preferences. A poor body image may hinder successful breastfeeding or even prevent any attempt. An antenatal teacher may not be able to bring about a major psychological change, but by encouraging positive attitudes and fostering self-confidence may be able to promote change. Partners can have an influence on decision-making and on ultimate success. The partner may be enthusiastic about breastfeeding or very much against it, but if the woman and her partner are at odds, differences may need to be resolved before feeding starts, if at all possible. A mother who wishes to breastfeed needs good information about the advantages and also how to play down what the partner may perceive as disadvantages. Equally, a mother whose partner wishes her to breastfeed against her own inclinations needs support to reinforce her decision. Breastfeeding begun under such circumstances is unlikely to succeed and may mar a mother's early contact with the baby. Mothers can be encouraged to discuss feeding with their partners if they have not already done so. A father may see the choice of feeding method as the mother's decision alone. He may later be upset by feelings of jealousy, because she is doing something for his son or daughter that he is unable to do, or perhaps may feel resentment against the baby for taking over breasts that were part of lovemaking.

The choice has frequently been made by the time antenatal classes are commenced, but a discussion of the advantages and disadvantages of both methods can help the waverers and may revise a decision that was made without much consideration. Criticizing a client's decision may undermine her confidence, either in herself or the people she regards as her mentors and upon whom she relies for support and security. Such an effect is not helpful. Midwives have a fine line to tread, promoting a positive attitude to breastfeeding while not inducing guilt in those who choose or who are constrained, for whatever reason, to bottlefeed. All mothers deserve our whole-hearted support.

(b) ADVANTAGES AND DISADVANTAGES OF FEEDING METHODS

The value of breast milk as a food for babies has been discussed and investigated by a wide range of people both

Baby Care and Feeding

from a scientific and an emotional point of view. When confronted with babies who seem contented and healthy when fed on modern formula milks, the specific advantages of breast milk may not be apparent to mothers. Milk is species-specific, each species producing milk with its constituents fulfilling the growth and energy requirements of the young.[1] The exact suitability of breast milk as a food for the human infant cannot be ignored. Modern societies may have expectations of scientists' ability 'to come up with the right answer', and yet in spite of improvements in infant formulae, doubts are still raised. For example, there is the question of aluminium levels and their potential as a cause of Alzheimer's disease.[2,3]

One factor which deserves serious consideration is the immunological significance of breast milk. The mother does not necessarily want or need to have detailed knowledge of immunoglobulins, lactoferrin, lysosome and the bifidus factor.[4] What will be useful is enough information for her to understand how the baby is unable to resist infection in the same way as an adult does. Sensible hygiene measures are not the only means of avoiding disease in the baby. Equally important are the factors in breast milk which fight pathogens and aid the development of the baby's own defence system. Illnesses in breastfed babies are often less severe than in bottlefed babies. In an age of antibiotics it is easy to be lulled into a false sense of security, devaluing the role of breast milk in combating not only bacterial but also viral infections.[5] Mothers often say, 'The milk hasn't come in yet, it's *only* colostrum', not realizing the value of the high levels of immunoglobulins in colostrum.[6] A mother may be concerned where there is a family history of an atopic disease such as eczema, asthma or hayfever. It is possible that allergens in formula milk may sensitize a susceptible infant, especially when given early in life, while the infant's own immune system is still immature.[7] Research continues in this field and breastfeeding cannot be regarded as a guarantee against atopic disease.

Baby Care and Feeding

Mothers sometimes ask questions about the possible danger to babies of chemicals polluting breast milk. Knowledge of this subject is far from complete. One study acknowledges the difficulty of assessing the potential risk, but feels the danger to babies from environmental chemicals is small. There are recorded cases where babies have suffered when mothers have been exposed to harmful chemicals in the course of their occupation.[8]

While research into bonding has looked more at general contact between mother and baby, mothers who have happily breastfed will testify to the very special close feeling engendered by breastfeeding. Breastfeeding a baby can also be a real sensual pleasure.

In a discussion on the relative convenience of feeding methods, opinions will vary according to the decision already made by the individual group members. A sharing of ideas can be useful to encourage clients to think about factors not previously considered. For example, a breastfeeding mother does not have to concern herself with shopping for supplies of formula, and teats and containers do not wear out! Making up feeds takes time and bottles of feed are one more thing that has to be remembered and carried when going out. However, a description of the joys of breastfeeding in bed at night is unlikely to change the mind of a bottlefeeder whose priorities include someone else being able to feed the baby.

Cost may or may not be of importance to your clients, but formula milk is expensive. Where financial resources are limited the baby's interests are best served by giving adequate nutrition to the mother. Not only does the baby have all the advantages of breast milk, but also lactation is a very energy-efficient process.[9]

Mothers are concerned about the effect of breastfeeding on their figures and an antenatal teacher needs to be able to give advice and reassurance. Few women notice a great difference in the size and shape of their breasts after breastfeeding. Some firmness may be lost but it is usually only after

Baby Care and Feeding

bearing several children, coupled with poor support of heavy breasts, that any appreciable change is noticed.

Body image and cultural traditions will affect a woman's attitude to breastfeeding in the presence of others. If she perceives this as a problem, it may prevent her breastfeeding. Neither the woman who is prepared to breastfeed anywhere no matter who is present, nor the woman who will only allow the presence of, at most, a close female relative, should be made to feel they are in any way wrong or odd. This must be a personal decision. The more modest or shy mothers can be given practical tips about suitable clothing if they have to feed in public. They may fail to realize how little of their body needs to be exposed to anyone but the baby!

Sharing the feeding of the baby with her partner may be a consideration. The partner may wish to be fully involved with caring for his baby and this may be a positive reason for choosing to bottlefeed. This is a decision which should be made with full knowledge of the advantages of breast milk, but in imparting this knowledge the antenatal teacher should be wary of making him feel selfish if the decision to bottlefeed is adhered to. Sharing the work (as opposed to the pleasures) of feeding, with partner or family, allowing the mother to do other work or socialize, may also be used as a reason for deciding to bottlefeed.

The need to return to work soon after the birth may be given as a reason for bottlefeeding. If you can explain the benefits of even a short period of breastfeeding, a mother may be prepared to give her baby the breast for that limited time, possibly continuing to breastfeed after her return to work, if this is practical (see below).

The mother's medical status may cause concern.[10] Conditions which preclude breastfeeding are not common; alternatives to harmful drugs can often be found. If the mother is sufficiently motivated, the physician can usually find a way. However, she may need your support and encouragement to put her case to her doctor. Equally, she may need your

Baby Care and Feeding

support if the answer has to be 'no' to breastfeeding – where lactation would put too great a strain on a mother's body or when the course of a disease would be adversely affected. The management of mothers with AIDS is likely to change as knowledge of the disease increases and current advice regarding breastfeeding should be sought. It is possible the infection can be transmitted via breast milk, but the advantages may outweigh the risk.

(c) THEORY AND PRACTICE OF BREASTFEEDING

A sound, though not necessarily highly detailed, knowledge of the anatomy and physiology of the breast and lactation will aid a mother in the establishment and maintenance of an adequate milk supply. She will have observed changes in her breasts during pregnancy. These observations can be used to begin a discussion on feeding. Despite an increase in size, those women with small breasts often doubt their ability to make enough milk. Size has nothing to do with efficiency: the non-pregnant breast is mostly fat and women with very small breasts have adequate glandular tissue and can lactate well. The appearance of Montgomery's tubercles may have been noticed. After mentioning this you could go on to discuss nipples, their preparation, care and possible associated difficulties. Although there are many traditional techniques for preparing nipples for feeding, none have been demonstrated under research conditions to be of benefit.[11] Montgomery's tubercles will produce adequate lubrication if this is not negated with the excessive use of such drying agents as soap, and no mechanical or topical preparation is effective in preventing soreness. The mother will be better prepared to fix the baby on the breast if she understands the anatomical principles of correct feeding techniques.[12] Nipple soreness can be avoided and healing enhanced if the baby is positioned correctly on the breast. Nipple shape and size is variable, the appearance of nipples having little to do with

Baby Care and Feeding

their efficiency. While in practice some difficulties may be experienced, it is more beneficial to a mother's confidence not to emphasize such difficulties. Think about whether it may be best to work on the principle that a baby will manage with whatever his mother has got. You can give clients some practical advice. You may feel it is appropriate to teach clients the way to test the protractability of their nipples (bearing in mind that this will increase as pregnancy advances), and either advise those who believe they have a problem or refer them to their own midwife for reassurance. The wearing of breast shells in pregnancy to improve nipple shape is advocated by some midwives, although their usefulness has not been proved by controlled trials. In class you can discuss methods that can be employed after the birth to cope with difficult nipples, use of nipple shields, breast pumps and, most important, skilled help from a midwife. The most helpful attitude antenatally is to acknowledge that problems may exist but leave the clients with a positive feeling that they can be overcome.

Some knowledge of the hormonal control of milk production and ejection can be of practical use to clients.[13] Understanding the role of prolactin and how its production can be improved by increasing the frequency and total length of sucking time will help them to maintain supply. Stress may inhibit oxytocin release and knowledge of this can enable them to attempt to avoid adverse conditions.[14]

Breastfeeding may be one factor that has an influence on the couple's sex life after the birth (see Chapters 4 and 9). The dual role of breasts in infant feeding and lovemaking can cause some concern. A couple may need to resolve conflicting feelings. A father may feel that while functioning as providers of nourishment for the baby, they can play no part in lovemaking. The mother, for reasons of physical discomfort, may not want her breasts touched. A couple may be grateful for the advice to feed the baby before lovemaking. This should stop a hungry baby disturbing them and prevents

Baby Care and Feeding

the excessive leaking of milk when oxytocin is released. Knowledge of the link between oxytocin release and sexual arousal may avoid concern or even guilt should the latter occur when the baby is feeding.

The most important factors in the establishment of successful breastfeeding apart from the mother's commitment are:

An early start.[15]
Proper fixing of the baby on the breast.[16]
No restrictions on duration and frequency of feeds.[17,18,19,20]
Skilled help when necessary.[21]

Think what you can do antenatally to assist the process. If mothers know the importance of an early start, they may be more eager to try, even though they may be tired immediately after labour. Nevertheless, care should be taken not to imply that missing an early start means failure. If you have doubts about the commitment to breastfeeding on the labour ward where your clients will deliver, tell the mothers to ask for help.

To fix a baby on the breast a mother may need no more than a willing baby placed in close proximity. However, it does not always happen as easily as that. An understanding of breast anatomy will help a mother to know when her baby is feeding correctly. Since babies need to open their mouth wide to take the breast, knowledge of the rooting reflex will aid the mother. Practical tips about getting the baby and herself into a comfortable and suitable position will be useful.

It is to be hoped that no restrictions will be placed on timing and duration of feeds, but if this does happen, a mother who has learnt the principles of lactation will be more able to resist bad advice, whoever it comes from. You may have no influence on the help available after birth but you can encourage clients to ask for help whenever and for

Baby Care and Feeding

as long as they feel they need it.

A mother may receive advice from many sources about what and what not to eat while breastfeeding. Much of what she may be told will be based on 'old wives' tales'. The ideal diet for breastfeeding is one which the mother enjoys and allows her to produce an adequate quantity of milk. This will vary considerably. You may feel it necessary to encourage a client to increase the variety of foods in her diet or to reduce the amount of 'empty calories' she consumes. In lactation the number of calories needed to produce a given quantity of milk is not as great as the theoretical calculation would suggest, since the body adapts its metabolism and becomes more energy-efficient (see note 9). The fat stores laid down in pregnancy are also made use of at this time. Appetite will often regulate food intake appropriately. Many mothers find they need a drink and a snack beside them when they sit down to feed, because breastfeeding makes them hungry and thirsty. If lactation and appetite are poor, then advice about increasing intake may be useful. Increasing fluid intake beyond the mother's thirst has not been shown to improve milk supply.[22] Breastfeeding mothers cite many different foods as producing unwanted effects in their babies, such as colic and diarrhoea. These appear to be individual reactions or even coincidental to food intake. While avoiding over-indulgence in any one food seems sensible, there is no evidence to support the banning of any particular foods to every breastfeeding mother. Allergic reactions to foods in the mother's diet are possible and if suspected, the mother should seek the advice of a paediatrican. One piece of useful information for clients is to tell them about the large number of bright yellow loose stools which the baby may pass when the milk first comes in. These are often seen as abnormal and blamed on 'something I ate', instead of the normal result of an increase in breast milk.

Losing excess weight gained in pregnancy is often of concern to mothers. Strict dieting is likely to reduce milk supply[23] and the body will use those fat stores during lactation, so making dieting unnecessary. You could remind mothers to avoid the foods which are high in calories but relatively low in nutritional value. They can diet more strictly, if necessary, once breastfeeding is finished.

The advice about alcohol, tobacco and drugs during breastfeeding differs little from advice given in pregnancy. Alcohol is best avoided or kept at a low level of intake, as it passes through into breast milk. Concentrations in milk are approximate to those in plasma and also decrease at similar rates. The baby's relatively immature liver is being asked to deal with an unnecessary drug.[24] Large amounts of alcohol interfere with the milk ejection reflex. Maybe one glass of celebratory champagne, but not the whole bottle! A breastfeeding mother may comment that her baby slept better when she fed it after taking alcohol, but it is not to be recommended as a way to pacify a baby.

Toxic components in cigarette smoke are a potential hazard to the baby. Nicotine reaches greater concentrations in breast milk than in the mother's blood. The level in the milk when the baby feeds will depend on the number of cigarettes smoked per day and the length of time since the last cigarette was smoked. The highest level will be reached immediately after smoking.[25]

Most drugs will pass into the milk and most will have no adverse effects on the baby, but caution is sensible.[26] Suggest that the mother consults the pharmacist when buying medicines over the counter, and reminds her general practitioner that she is breastfeeding when drugs are being prescribed.

A well-designed and properly fitting nursing bra will add greatly to comfort and convenience when breastfeeding. Some useful pointers when choosing a bra are: cups that not only fit well but also support the upper half of the breast (a low-cut lacy cup may look glamorous but will not be comfortable if a full breast is falling out over the top); cups should support but not flatten the breast, and a seam which cuts

Baby Care and Feeding

across the nipple may cause discomfort; a wide band under the bust is more comfortable, as are wide straps, especially if the breasts are very large and heavy. There are many styles of opening in nursing bras. Some have centrally placed hooks and eyes, but mothers may prefer designs which allow one-handed operation – zips or clips which hold a flap in place. Good fitting is important. You may be able to discover which local shops give you a good service and you may have a National Childbirth Trust bra fitter in your area. Mothers may be reluctant to spend a lot of money on bras before the birth, not being sure if it will be the correct size. You could suggest they are fitted with at least one in the last few weeks before they give birth. It will then be easy to ask someone to buy them another one or two after the birth, adjusting the size if necessary. When the milk comes in they will appreciate a comfortable bra and it is a very difficult time for a mother to either go and buy or be fitted for a bra. If the mother sends someone else to buy a bra when she has no idea what is needed, she is unlikely to get a well-fitting one.

Mothers may have unrealistic expectations of feeding patterns and it can be useful to prepare them for some possibilities. A mother should be reassured that a baby who is sleepy and feeds infrequently for a day or two after birth is behaving normally. It can then come as a shock if, on day three and four, her 'good' baby suddenly demands feeds every hour, but this is also normal and does not mean she has an inadequate supply. Prolactin response to suckling has been shown to be greater at night.[27] This is one reason why the successful establishment of breastfeeding is enhanced by 'round the clock' demand feeding and mothers should be encouraged to be prepared to feed at night. If in the antenatal period you can help them to see this as necessary and desirable, it may be easier for them to accept a different pattern of sleep. Mothers may believe it necessary to feed a baby from both breasts at every feed and impose a time

Baby Care and Feeding

limit on the first breast, thus possibly denying the baby the high-calorie hind milk.[28,29]

It can be useful if the mothers are aware of some of the common problems which may occur with feeding in the early days. A mother may experience difficulty in fixing the baby on the breast or may experience pain when the baby sucks. In either case she needs the help of a midwife. You can encourage her to ask for help and keep asking until she gets it right. She should not feel she is incompetent or stupid if she needs more help than her neighbour. Vascular engorgement may cause discomfort around two to four days after the birth but mothers can be reassured it is only temporary. Milk engorgement can usually be avoided if the baby is allowed unrestricted access to the breasts, and this is one reason why night feeding should be encouraged.

Mothers are less likely to worry about whether or not they have an adequate supply of milk if they understand how lactation is maintained. They will not then fall into the trap of offering a supplementary feed when a baby demands feeds more frequently, but allow the baby to feed more often and so increase the supply. It is also useful for mothers to know how tiredness may affect supply.

Mothers can be assured that infections in themselves will rarely mean that breastfeeding should be discontinued. Rather, a baby is protected by the immune mechanisms in the mother, which provide immunity via the milk.[30]

(d) THEORY AND PRACTICE OF BOTTLEFEEDING

Preparations for bottlefeeding include deciding which formula to use, which bottles and teats to buy, and how to sterilize the equipment.

The baby milk formulae on sale in this country conform to DHSS standards, so mothers can have the confidence of knowing that, as far as present knowledge extends, any of the milks are suitable.[31] Do you know which choice she will

Baby Care and Feeding

be offered in the hospital? There are only minor differences between the different brands but some differences may have significance for clients. For example, vegetarian, Jewish, Muslim or Hindu mothers may not be happy to use a milk containing beef fat, (SMA). Mothers with allergies, or vegan mothers, may prefer to use a formula not based on cow's milk. Soy-based milks are not without their problems and it is sensible for clients to seek the advice of a paediatrician before feeding a baby on one of these formulae. You could also discuss the relative merits of methods of sterilizing bottles. Chemical cold-water sterilizing is a common and efficient method if carried out according to instructions. This is a point which could be made in class. Boiling is used less than previously, but it is effective. There is a steam sterilizer designed for domestic use, but it is expensive, although efficient and quick to operate. You may think it useful to discuss different bottle and teat designs. Most babies will accept any design of teat, but others may feed better with a 'natural' shape or 'anti-colic' teat. Disposable bottles are now available; these may work out more expensive, but this may be outweighed by the convenience factor. Many hospitals will encourage babies to bottlefeed on demand rather than to a strict regime. Do you know how mothers will be advised in your area? Will lactation be suppressed pharmacologically or naturally? A supportive bra will be especially useful during natural suppression, if the breasts become full and heavy.

(e) OTHER PRACTICAL FEEDING CONSIDERATIONS

Think about what advice you will give mothers about 'winding' a baby after feeds. Breastfed babies usually swallow less air with feeds than bottlefeeders. Patting or rubbing a baby's back too vigorously is not necessary and may disturb a baby who is content and relaxed after a feed. Mothers may be unprepared for the 'posseting' which may occur after feeds

Baby Care and Feeding

and interpret it as vomiting and a cause for concern.

Consider whether you should discuss weaning. Mothers may ask when they should stop breastfeeding. There is no correct length of time; babies should be given either breast milk or a baby milk formula for at least six months. 'Doorstep' milk should not be given before six months and some authorities believe leaving the changeover until nine months or a year is advantageous.[32] It may seem early to discuss starting a baby on solid food but mothers may have questions about when it should be tried. Breastfeeding older babies may cause concern to mothers, either because they wish to finish and the baby does not, or because there is pressure to give up from family or others. The experience of other mothers can be a useful resource.[33]

It may be useful to ask clients to consider sources of help with feeding when they return home. The midwife is the obvious person to give advice at first, but after she has completed her care, who then? The health visitor will be available but lay resources should not be ignored. The mother's own family and circle of friends may possess a large amount of experience in feeding babies. The organizations which support breastfeeding mothers – the National Childbirth Trust, Association of Breastfeeding Mothers and La Leche League – can give advice and also valuable social contact (See Appendix 1).

Returning to work may pose problems with feeding. If a mother is breastfeeding happily, she does not necessarily need to make a complete change to bottlefeeding. Jobs which will accommodate a breastfeeding baby on the premises may be few, but you could suggest the mother considers the alternatives. She could breastfeed when she is at home and allow the baby to have formula milk when she is not. It may be difficult to maintain an adequate supply under such conditions, but she should continue as long as possible, if she is happy to do so. She could express at work and take the milk home for the next day's feeds. She will need access

Baby Care and Feeding

to a refrigerator to store the milk during the day. Many mothers have found combining work and breastfeeding a practical proposition when given sensible advice.[34]

(f) CARE OF THE BABY BY THE MOTHER

When you discuss caring for the baby is may be useful to encourage clients to voice their feelings, which may include feelings of inadequacy. New mothers sometimes believe they are expected instinctively to know how to care for a baby. They feel far from confident and yet reluctant to admit this. It can be helpful if you give clients the opportunity to share such feelings with others.

You can help to build up their confidence by drawing out the knowledge they do have. For example they may say they do not know how much clothing they should put on their baby. If you ask them to think about factors such as weather conditions and room temperature and how warm or cold they feel, they can understand how they would arrive

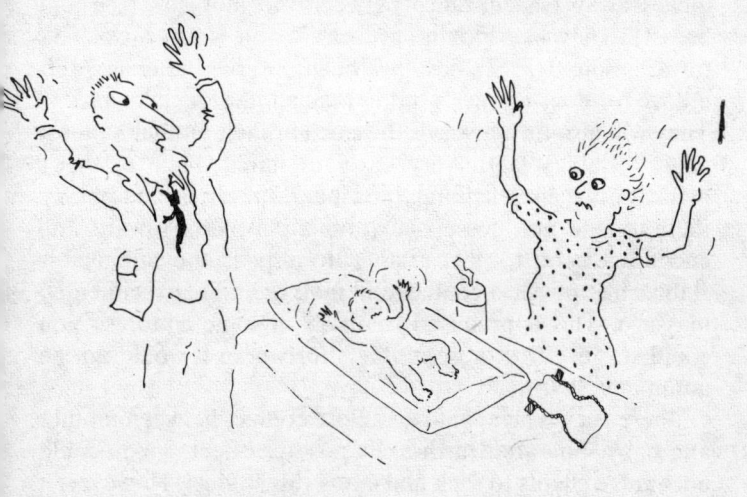

You will encounter the startle reflex

Baby Care and Feeding

at a common sense answer. You can add some more information if necessary, such as, to touch the body rather than extremities when feeling a baby to see how warm or cold it is, or remembering to put a hat on because of the considerable heat loss which can occur from the head.

The capabilities of a newborn infant will provide material for a useful and interesting discussion. Although many mothers are well informed, a baby's sense of sight, hearing, touch, smell and taste are far more acute than they often realize. Knowing this can encourage more interaction between mother and baby to the advantage of them both. A baby may spend very little time awake in the first few days, especially if it has received drugs via the placenta during labour. You could encourage mothers to make the most of the times when their babies are alert. This may happen naturally, but they will be more likely to attempt to communicate if they believe the baby is aware and able to respond. Eye contact between people is important for communication. Newborns focus best if the subject is nine to ten inches away (the distance between the mother's face and breast). They like looking at faces,[35] and will turn to look towards sounds.[36] Babies have been observed to show preference for their mother's rather than another female voice.[37] They will also turn towards the smell of their mother's breast milk.[38] Babies learn very early to mimic their mother's behaviour, such as smiling, blowing 'raspberries' and poking their tongue out. Response from a baby is a reward and encouragement to the mother to repeat the stimulus.[39] Babies like physical contact and mother and baby will enjoy massage. This is practised routinely in some cultures. You could suggest it to those mothers for whom it would not be automatic.[40,41]

There is evidence that early close contact between mother and baby soon after birth has a positive effect.[42] You could encourage clients to seek and enjoy this contact. However, it would be wrong to suggest the long-term relationship with

Baby Care and Feeding

her child would be harmed if this did not happen. The developing relationship between mother and baby may be assisted if the mother understands this is a gradual process not an instant bond. Babies need affection, security, consistency and stimulation. It would be helpful to ensure clients are aware of these positive factors.[43] Babies will interact with their mothers if they are given the opportunity to do so. But babies are different and it will help a mother if she realizes this. For example, babies need affection but vary in their appreciation of being cuddled.[44] The development of a positive emotional relationship between mother and baby may need no assistance, but when conditions are less than optimum the mother may need help and reassurance, for example, if she and her baby are separated because of illness or if her baby is difficult to feed or settle.

It is useful to discuss crying. Crying is one way a baby communicates with its mother and she can learn to interpret her baby's different cries. You could ask your clients to suggest the reasons why a baby cries and how a mother should respond. They may say hunger, pain or cold, but may not realize a baby can also be bored, lonely or frustrated.[45] What response is appropriate depends on the reason. At first a mother may feel inadequate if she does not immediately know what her baby wants. If hunger is not the reason, as it often is in the early days, she can look for the other possible reasons. Often babies want contact with someone, being held or rocked, but are sometimes deprived of this because of a fear of 'spoiling' the child. Mothers can be discouraged from believing this; babies are more likely to be content if their needs are attended to than if they are left to cry.[46] Other means of calming a crying baby which may work are swaddling, or some sound, for example, womb sounds,[47] white noise, music or talking. Every mother has probably experienced an occasion when nothing would calm her baby. If she is unlucky, this can happen frequently, especially in the first three months. Regular, inconsolable crying is often

Baby Care and Feeding

attributed to colic. There does not seem to be a consensus of opinion about the cause or treatment of colic. Maureen Minchin offers some theories and possible management.[48] If her doctor has reassured her the baby is healthy, the mother needs support to get through this difficult time. There may be no apparent reason, although a difficult birth could be a possible cause.[49] Mothers may be helped by contact with other mothers in the same situation through organizations such as CRY-SIS and Meet-a-Mum (see Appendix 1).

It would be helpful if you knew what opportunities your clients will have for learning to care for their babies in the early days. The babies may stay by the bedside round the clock, or the hospital may have a policy of putting the babies in a nursery at certain times. If the mothers are given a choice about 'rooming in', what will you advise them to do? Being constantly with her baby will enable a mother to learn, but if she is exhausted through lack of sleep during labour or after, it may be helpful if midwives do care for the baby for a short while. Think about how the mothers, the hospital and you feel about babies in bed with mothers. In spite of fears about suffocating babies, there is no evidence that this is a problem.[50] It is an excellent way of keeping babies warm, of pacifying a crying baby and a comfortable and restful way of feeding at night. The only times when it could constitute a hazard to the baby are when the mother (or father) has taken alcohol or sleeping tablets, or is ill.

(g) CARE OF THE BABY BY THE MIDWIFE

Every mother wants the reassurance that her baby is well and healthy. You could describe the checks the midwife carries out soon after birth. Find out if they will be done in the presence of the mother. The appearance of a normal, newborn infant may not be what the mother expects. You may feel it appropriate to point out some features which may cause concern, such as moulding of the head or birth marks.

Baby Care and Feeding

You could explain the daily checks on the baby by the midwife. Many mothers know babies lose weight after birth, but still need reassurance that the loss is within normal limits. The appearance and consistency of stools requires explanation; in particular the mothers may need convincing that the normal looseness of a breastfed baby's stools is not diarrhoea. The stump of the umbilical cord worries many mothers, fearing they will hurt the baby if they touch it or the baby will bleed if they knock it off. Some blood tests are routine, such as the Guthrie test. It will be helpful if clients could have an explanation of the reasons for any tests.

(h) CARE OF THE BABY BY THE PAEDIATRICIAN

You could tell the mothers about the routine paediatric care the baby will receive. Examinations may be carried out in the presence of the mother. An explanation of the examination done by the paediatrician can help the mother understand why the tests are done and what they can tell us about the baby. Most clients will have some knowledge of the primitive reflexes, being aware that a baby will grasp, root and suck. You could go on to discuss the less well-known Moro and stepping reflexes. You will need to judge how much detail they want about the physical examination. The test for congenital dislocation of the hip deserves some explanation; it can often cause the mother distress because the baby sometimes seems to be in pain as it is being done. She may not remember everything that is discussed, but you can encourage her to ask for explanations from the paediatrician at the time.

Think what you will tell clients about what will happen if something is wrong with the baby. If mothers feel safe and secure in the environment of the group, many will, given the opportunity, discuss worries about the safety and health of the baby. You will not be able to ensure they have no worries but a sharing of concern may help clients. What a midwife

Baby Care and Feeding

perceives as a normal occurrence or a minor problem may cause great distress. You cannot hope to prepare them for everything that may happen but some discussion of common problems can be useful. A baby who is cold can often be warmed sufficiently, well-wrapped in a warm room or put in bed with mother, but an uninformed mother may be upset if the baby has to go into an incubator. Skin rashes and 'sticky' eyes may look spectacular but need only simple treatment, or none at all. Understanding of why some babies may be at risk from low blood-sugar and of the routine tests carried out after birth can reassure a mother, should this happen. Jaundice in the first week of life requires some explanation. It is most likely to be physiological and may or may not need treatment. If phototherapy is required, this may be done on the postnatal ward or may mean separation of mother and baby if treatment is done on the neonatal unit.

Consider whether you will raise the possibility of more serious problems or wait for mothers to ask. You could give information about congenital abnormalities or demonstrate a willingness to discuss the subject if clients wish. The degree of distress a mother exhibits when confronted with an abnormality in her baby is not necessarily related to its severity. It may be influenced by an emotional reaction or by lack of knowledge. The former you can probably do little about but you may be able to increase her knowledge if she is willing to learn.

The policies of caring for the premature infant could be discussed. It may be helpful if you know what criteria the paediatricians use for deciding whether a small baby remains with the mother or is cared for on a neonatal unit. If a client is expecting twins or there is another reason for believing she is likely to give birth to a premature baby, a visit to the neonatal unit could prepare a mother to cope better with the stress of the experience. The news that twins are expected is often greeted with 'Oh how lovely', but is it always a joy? Two babies at once can strain a family's physical, emotional

Baby Care and Feeding

and financial resources and acknowledgement of this, with practical hints for managing twins, may be appreciated. Other mothers of twins may be best source of advice. You could put clients in touch with the Twins and Multiple Births Association (TAMBA) (see Appendix 1).

(i)...

Can you think of anything else clients may need to know or want to know?

4 How Will You Teach?

A discussion on feeding babies is likely to bring out many different opinions. Sharing ideas can help the clients increase their knowledge and clarify their feelings. You will be able to correct any misinformation.

You may feel there are some things you must tell them, for example, that it is dangerous to leave a baby lying flat on its back because of the risk of inhalation of vomit. But if you can do it in a way that makes them think, the learning is more thorough. Many may already know that it is a dangerous practice – you could ask them to explain why they believe it. If clients do not know, you could show them the relative positions of oesophagus and trachea and then ask them to imagine what will happen if the baby vomits when lying supine.

You could demonstrate comfortable positions for feeding babies. You could demonstrate how to fix a baby on to the breast correctly, using visual aids. A demonstration of how to make a feed and sterilize equipment could be done antenatally, but it may be better to leave this until after the birth, since it is unlikely that clients will remember the details of such instruction. You may feel it is appropriate to demonstrate some practical skills: how to change a nappy, how to

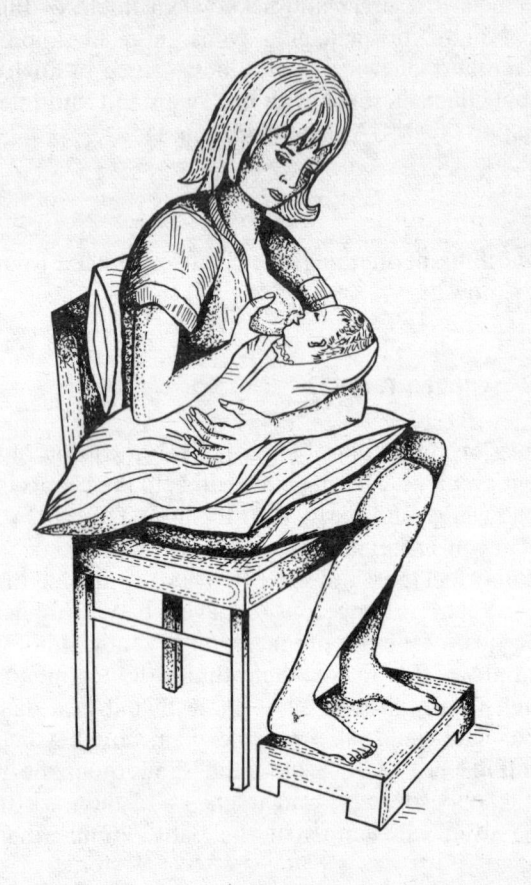

Fig. 8.1 A comfortable position for feeding

'top and tail' or bath a baby. The mothers are more likely to learn these skills postnatally, especially if they have no opportunity to practise in the antenatal period. However, if you bath a baby, it will be a chance for them to have a really good look at a newborn baby and you will be able to point out some of the normal features of the newborn. They may

Baby Care and Feeding

then be prompted to ask questions. Consider whether bathing a doll is of value.

In discussions you may be able to involve experienced mothers either from within the group or specially invited, or perhaps a recently delivered mother who can talk about how she is learning her mothering skills.

A visit to the postnatal ward and a neonatal unit may be possible.

5 What Aids Will You Use?

A film or video showing mothers discussing feelings, practicalities and problems can be useful, giving a wide range of opinions and experiences.

Various aids could be used to demonstrate correct breastfeeding technique, including pictures and videos. A breastfeeding mother in class can act as an excellent aid, if this is acceptable to the mother and the group. Clients will have the opportunity to question her, which cannot happen with a video. It will, however, be only one person's experience.

A film or video depicting a newborn's capabilities, or showing an examination by a paediatrician, may be useful.

Consider if it would be possible to have a paediatrician examining a baby in the class.

Other aids to consider: pictures of breast anatomy and how a baby fixes and feeds on the breast, visual illustration of 'let down' reflex, nursing bras, bottles and sterilizers.

6 Trigger Questions to Stimulate Discussion

What advantages (or disadvantages) do you see in breastfeeding?
What advantages (or disadvantages) do you see in bottlefeeding?

Baby Care and Feeding

How would you feel about feeding in the park or in front of a male relative?
What do you expect breastfeeding to do to your figure?
What changes have you noticed in your breasts since you became pregnant?
If you believe you don't have enough breast milk for your baby, what can you do?
Has anyone told you about foods you should not eat when you are breastfeeding?
Have friends told you which are the best bottles/teats/formula milks?
What have friends or relatives told you about problems with feeding?
Have you held a newborn baby?
  How did you feel?
What do you think a baby needs most of all?
What do you know about how a newborn baby sees/smells?

7 How Will You Know When You Have Done It?

Feedback in class will help you estimate how much knowledge has been taken in and how clients feel about caring for their babies. If you have the opportunity to observe them feeding and looking after their babies in the early days, this will help you to evaluate your teaching. Think about using a questionnaire in class or after birth to assess clients' learning. A reunion class may also provide feedback for you to assess client learning and evaluate your teaching.

Suggested Leaflets

From Health Education Authority:

How to Survive the First Week of Breastfeeding.
A Simple Guide to Bottle Feeding.

Baby Care and Feeding

From the National Childbirth Trust:

Thinking about breastfeeding.
Breastfeeding – a good start.
Breastfeeding – avoiding some of the problems.
Breastfeeding – not enough milk?
How to express and store breast milk.
Breastfeeding – too much milk?
Breastfeeding if your baby needs special care.
Breastfeeding. (In English, Gujerati, Punjabi, Bengali, Hindi and Urdu.)

From La Leche League:

Beginning breastfeeding.

From Twins and Multiple Birth Association:

Arrival of Twins.
Breast Feeding Twins.
Bottle Feeding Twins.

References

1 Lawrence, R. A. (1985), *Breastfeeding. A Guide for the Medical Profession*, 2nd edn, C. V. Mosby, St Louis, pp. 65–116.
2 Birchall, J. D. and Chappell, J. S. (1988), 'Aluminium, chemical physiology and Alzheimer's disease', *The Lancet*, vol. 2, 29 October, pp. 1008–1010.
3 Freundlich, M., Zilleruelo, G., Abitbol, C., Strauss, J., Faugere, M. C. and Malluche, H. H. (1985), 'Infant formula as a cause of aluminium toxicity in neonatal uraemia', *The Lancet*, vol. 2, 7 September, pp. 527–9.
4 Lawrence, R. A., *Breastfeeding. A Guide for the Medical Profession*, pp. 117–40.
5 Ibid., p. 136.
6 Ibid., pp. 125–7.
7 Ibid., pp. 399–407.

Baby Care and Feeding

8   Rogan, W. J., Bagniewska, A. and Damstra, T. (1980), 'Pollutants in breast milk', *New England Journal of Medicine*, vol. 302, no. 26, pp. 1450–3.

9   Illingworth, P. J., Jung, R. T., Howie, P. W., Leslie, P. and Isles, T. E. (1986), 'Diminution in energy expenditure during lactation', *British Medical Journal*, vol. 292, pp. 437–41.

10 Lawrence, *Breastfeeding. A Guide for the Medical Profession*, pp. 357–98.

11 (1986) *Successful Breastfeeding. A Practical Guide for Midwives*, The Royal College of Midwives, (1988), pp. 50–2.

12 Woolridge, M. W., 'The "anatomy" of infant sucking', *Midwifery*, vol. 2, pp. 164–71.

13 McNeilly, A. S., Robinson, I. C. A., Houston, M. J. and Howie, P. W. (1983), 'Release of oxytocin and prolactin in response to suckling', *British Medical Journal*, vol. 286, pp. 257–9.

14 Lawrence, *Breastfeeding. A Guide for the Medical Profession*, pp. 198–9.

15 Salariya, E. M., Easton, P. M. and Cater, J. I. (1978), 'Duration of feeding after early initiation and frequent feeding', *The Lancet*, vol. 2, pp. 1141–3.

16 The Royal College of Midwives, *Successful Breastfeeding. A Practical Guide for Midwives*, pp. 9–12; 17–27.

17 De Carvalho, M., Robertson, S., Friedman, A. and Klaus, M. (1983), 'Effect of frequent breastfeeding on early milk production and infant weight gain', *Paediatrics*, vol. 72, no. 3, September, pp. 307–11.

18 Howie, P. W., Houston, M. J., Cook, A., Smart, L., McArdle, T. and McNeilly, A. S. (1981), 'How long should a breast feed last?' *Early Human Development*, vol. 5, pp. 71–7.

19 Slaven, S. and Harvey, D. (1981), 'Unlimited suckling time improves breastfeeding', *The Lancet*, vol. 1, 14 February, pp. 392–3.

20 Woolridge, M. W., Baum, J. D. and Drewett, R. F. (1982), 'Individual patterns of milk intake during breast feeding', *Early Human Development*, vol. 7, pp. 265–72.

21 The Royal College of Midwives, *Successful Breastfeeding. A Practical Guide for Midwives*, pp. 29–41.

22 Dusdieker, L. B., Booth, B. M., Stumbo, P. J. and Eichenberger, J. M. (1985), 'Effect of supplemental fluids on human milk production', *Journal of Paediatrics*, vol. 106, no. 2, pp. 207–11.

23 Crawford, M. A., Laurance, B. M. and Munhambo, A. E. (1977), 'Breast Feeding and Human Milk Composition', *The Lancet*, vol. 1, 8 January, pp. 99–100.

24 Redetski, H. M. (1981), 'Alcohol'. In: *Drugs in Breast Milk*, Wilson, J. T. (ed), MTP Press Ltd, pp. 46–9.

Baby Care and Feeding

25 Steldinger, R. and Luck, W. (1988), 'Half lives of nicotine in milk of smoking mothers: implications for nursing', *Journal of Perinatal Medicine*, vol. 16, pp. 261–2.

26 Lewis, P. J. and Hurden, E. L. (1987), 'Breast feeding and drug treatment'. In: *Drugs and Pregnancy*, Hawkins, D. F. (ed), Churchill Livingstone, Edinburgh, pp. 304–32.

27 Glasier, A. S., McNeilly, A. S. and Howie, P. W. (1984), 'The prolactin response to suckling', *Clinical Endocrinology*, vol. 21, pp. 109–116.

28 Lawrence, *Breastfeeding. A Guide for the Medical Profession*, p. 198.

29 Hytten, F. E. (1954), 'Clinical and chemical studies in human lactation', *British Medical Journal*, vol. 1, 23 January, pp. 175–82.

30 Howie, P. W. (1985), 'Breast feeding – a new understanding', *Midwives Chronicle*, Vol. 98, no. 1170, July, pp. 184–92.

31 DHSS, *Present day Practice in Infant Feeding. Third Report*, Report on Health and Social Subjects no. 32, HMSO, London.

32 Ibid., p. 31.

33 Fage, J., Macwhinnie, J. and Osmotherly, V. (1983), *Nursing Beyond One*, National Childbirth Trust, London.

34 Price, A. and Bamford, N. (1984), *The Breastfeeding Guide for the Working Woman*, Century, London.

35 Fantz, R. L. (1963), 'Pattern vision in newborn infants', *Science*, vol. 140, pp. 296–7.

36 Wertheimer, M. (1961), 'Psychomotor co-ordination of auditory-visual space at birth', *Science*, vol. 134, p. 1692.

37 DeCaspar, A. J. and Fifer, W. P. (1980), 'Of human bonding: newborns prefer their mothers' voices', *Science*, vol. 208, 6 June, pp. 1174–6.

38 Macfarlane, A. (1977), *The Psychology of Childbirth*, Fontana/Open Books, Glasgow, pp. 84–6.

39 Meltzoff, A. N. and Moore, M. K. (1977), 'Facial and manual imitation by human neonates', *Science*, vol. 198, pp. 75–7.

40 Heinl, T. (1982), *The Baby Massage Book*, Coventure, London.

41 Walker, P. (1986), *Baby Relax. A Parents' Guide to Baby Massage and Baby Gymnastics*, Unwin, London.

42 Macfarlane, *The Psychology of Childbirth*, pp. 94–103.

43 Prince, J. and Adams, M. E. (1987), *The Psychology of Childbirth. An Introduction for Mothers and Midwives*, 2nd edn, Churchill Livingstone, Edinburgh, pp. 162–9.

44 Ibid., pp. 18–20.

45 Davies, M. D., Lloyd, E. and Scheffler, A. (1987), *Baby Language*, Unwin, London, pp. 40–7.

46 Dunn, J. (1982), *Distress and Comfort*, Fontana/Open Books, Glasgow, pp. 62–4.

47 Callis, P. M. (1984), 'The testing and comparison of the intra-uterine

sound against other methods for calming babies', *Midwives Chronicle*, vol. 97, no. 1161, October, pp. 336–8.
48 Minchin, M. (1985), *Breastfeeding Matters*, Allen and Unwin, Australia.
49 Dunn, J., *Distress and Comfort*, pp. 16–18.
50 The Royal College of Midwives, *Successful Breastfeeding. A Practical Guide for Midwives*, p. 36.

Further Reading

Bryan, E. (1983), *The Nature and Nurture of Twins*, Baillière Tindall, London.

Bryan, E. (1984), *Twins in the Family – A Parents' Guide*, Constable, London.

Clegg, A. and Woollett, A. (1983), *Twins from Conception to Five Years*, Century, London.

Douglas, J. and Richman, N. (1984), *My Child Won't Sleep*, Penguin, Harmondsworth.

Glover, B. and Hodson, C. (1985), *You and Your Premature Baby*, Sheldon, London.

Palmer, G. (1988), *The Politics of Breastfeeding*, Pandora, London.

Redshaw, M. E., Rivers, R. P. A. and Rosenblatt, D. B. (1985), *Born Too Early. Special Care for Your Pre-term Baby*, Oxford University Press, Oxford.

Savage King, F. (1985), *Helping Mothers to Breast Feed*, African Medical and Research Foundation, Nairobi.

9
Life After Birth

Your clients may have thought little about how they will feel after the birth, while the hurdle of labour is still before them. For many, becoming a mother will be the biggest revolution in their lives. Think about how you can help them to cope with the changes in their lives so that they experience the minimum amount of trauma and the maximum amount of joy.

1 What Are Your Aims?

Clients will be able to:

Be prepared for the realities of parenthood.
Explore their feelings and resolve possible conflicts.
Discover the means to cope with practical and emotional problems of parenting.
Or . . . ?

Having your aims in mind,

2 What Are Your Objectives?

At the end of the session the mothers will be able to:

Recall the basic physiology of the puerperium.
Identify symptoms she should report to her midwife.

Life After Birth

Discuss possible emotional reactions she may experience.
Discuss how changing roles may affect the relationship with her partner.
Or . . .?

3 What Will You Teach?

(a) PHYSICAL NEEDS AND CARE IN THE PUERPERIUM

Before the birth women may find it difficult to think about what their own needs will be after the birth. Physical and emotional feelings after birth may take a mother by surprise. An explanation of the changes taking place in a woman's body as it recovers from pregnancy and birth will help her to understand why the midwives make the routine observations of temperature, pulse and blood pressure, lochia and involution of the uterus, breasts, urinary and alimentary tracts, legs and perineum. She can be made aware of the blood test and the reason for haemoglobin estimation.

Knowledge of the physiology of the puerperium is also important in her own part in maintaining her health and comfort. You can encourage her to tell her midwife if her lochia seems heavy or she is loosing clots, if her perineum is painful or micturition causes a burning sensation. Mothers may not always complain of the aches and pains they perceive as minor. Care of the perineum, although supervised by a midwife, is to a great extent under the control of the mother herself. She needs to understand the importance of keeping it clean and dry. Consider if she knows what a bidet is and how to use one. Even in this affluent, modern world not everyone has seen one. If we assume knowledge, those women unfamiliar with this appliance may be too embarrassed to ask for an explanation. The hospital may provide sanitary towels or she may have to bring her own supply. She may not realize how frequently she may need to change her

Life After Birth

pads in the first days. Pain from a sutured perineum can mar the enjoyment of her baby in the first few days; you could teach her some simple remedies which may relieve it. Warm baths, ice packs, sitting on a ring cushion or pillow or lying down to feed her baby are a few suggestions. Find out what else the hospital can offer. Topical applications may be used. The physiotherapist may give ultrasound treatment. Some mothers may be reluctant to take analgesic tablets, believing them harmful to the baby if ingested through the breast milk, and will need reassurance. Bath additives are sometimes used. These are not of proven efficacy,[1] but the practice is common. Midwives are anxious to avoid any postnatal infection, but often face problems with ward hygiene. Lack of staff, cut-backs in finance, difficulties with cleaners can all cause standards to be lower than desired. If mothers are alerted to report any shortfall, they will protect their own interests.[2]

There may be hospital policies it would be useful for clients to know about. The baby may stay by the mother's bed all the time or may be taken into a nursery, either at her request or the midwife's suggestion. You could encourage mothers to think how they might feel about separation from their babies. A mother may be upset at the thought of being parted from her baby or relieved that the midwives will care for her baby so she is able to sleep. The work done by researchers on bonding has in some instances swung the pendulum so far the other way that instead of being forcibly separated from their babies in hospital, they are given no choice about having their babies constantly with them, thus reducing the opportunity to have the rest they so desperately need. Antenatally, mothers can be encouraged to find pleasure in early contact with their babies, but should not be made to feel guilt or regret if, because of their own disinclination or unavoidable separation, they miss the opportunity to spend time with their babies immediately after birth.[3] Clients may like to know the visiting hours in the

Life After Birth

hospital. Open visiting may be convenient for the visitors but tiring for the mothers. Consider introducing the idea antenatally that regulation of her visitors either by the mother or her immediate family may benefit her. Adequate rest is important for recovery and the establishment of breast-feeding, and the mother can be encouraged to make this one of her priorities. Waking a sleeping mother in the postnatal period should be prohibited. A hungry baby is the one exception.

Mothers with special needs should be prepared for their own situation. Mothers with a Rhesus negative blood group can be prepared for the anti-D injection if required. Where an elective Caesarean section is planned, advice about exercise, movement and comfort can be tailored to their requirements. Some information may be remembered after an emergency Caesarean is performed, but it is not realistic to expect all clients to remember this information. The prospect of caring for two or more babies can be daunting and other mothers who have done so are a valuable resource for

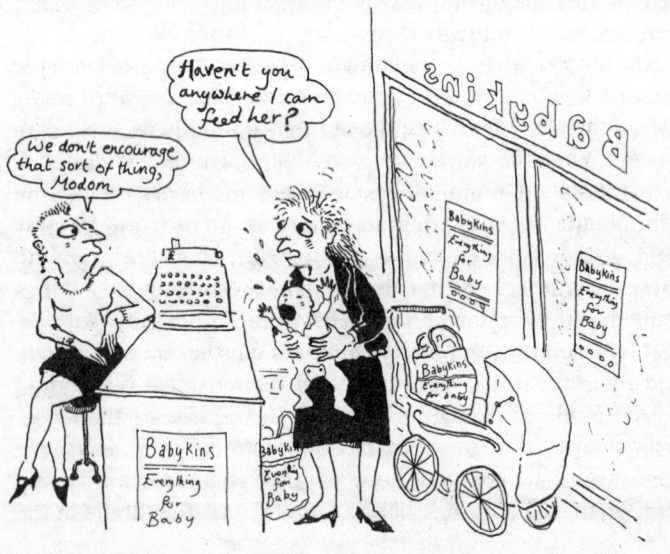

Life After Birth

clients. An occupational therapy department alerted before the birth may be able to offer suggestions to assist a physically disabled mother.

An understanding of how exercise can improve health and well-being may encourage mothers not only to exercise in hospital but also to continue at home. Mothers looking forward to a flat abdomen and wearing their jeans or other pre-pregnancy clothes can understand the need for exercising abdominal muscles. The necessity for exercising pelvic floor muscles may require more explanation. Immediately after the birth, exercising bruised, cut or torn muscles may seem to the mother undesirable, difficult or even impossible. An explanation of how increasing the blood flow through those muscles by exercise can reduce swelling and speed healing may encourage her. An inefficient pelvic floor leads to problems of stress incontinence and good teaching at this time can have long-term benefits for her health and happiness. Exercising leg muscles to improve circulation probably has less significance now, when mothers are ambulant soon after birth, but is helpful in the early days, especially when there are varicose veins or swollen ankles.

An obstetric physiotherapist may give mothers instruction in exercise after birth but, as every hospital does not have one on the staff, a midwife needs the knowledge to teach her clients. When talking antenatally about postnatal exercises it is not reasonable to expect mothers to remember instructions for a complete course; it is to be hoped instruction will take place after the birth. A few basic principles can be taught: start early, start gently, never do anything which causes strain, and do the exercises little and often. Abdominal exercises should be done lying supine on the bed with knees bent up – breathing out, pulling in the abdominal muscles, holding briefly before relaxing – doing this four times, several times a day. Ankle exercises can be done with the legs supported, for thirty seconds at a time, three or four times a day, flexing the ankles up and down, remembering

Life After Birth

that firm dorsiflexion is the more important action. Pelvic floor exercises (see page 77), to be effective, should be done four at a time, totalling two hundred times a day. Mothers often find this information startling, but if you can encourage them to associate this exercise with other routine daily activities, such as feeding the baby, urinating, washing up or answering the telephone, it become less of a chore. Perineal muscle function after childbirth is related to the amount of exercise before the event. Those women who do any form of regular exercise are more likely to have good pelvic floor tone and strength,[4] the importance of antenatal preparation should be emphasized.

(b) EMOTIONAL AND SEXUAL NEEDS IN THE PUERPERIUM

The emotional care of a newly delivered mother is as important as her physical needs. Preparation can help her to cope with the often labile and disturbing emotions of this period. The baby may be so much the centre of attention that the mother feels neglected. Ask her to think whether she expects to feel a rush of maternal affection the first time she looks at her baby. It can be an upsetting experience if this expectation is not fulfilled. It may help women to understand this if you ask them if they fell in love with their husband or boyfriend at first sight. Realization that development of a relationship with the baby can also take time can save the mother distress. Many have heard about 'the baby blues' and a discussion does help them to cope should they experience it. Eating the placenta has been suggested as a means of preventing postnatal depression. Although probably little practised, it may be an issue raised by your clients.[5] In an effort to prepare them to cope with problems after the birth we should beware of painting too black a picture. Mothers need reassurance they can do the job they were made for,[6] and we can bolster or help to

Life After Birth

destroy confidence by our attitudes in antenatal teaching.

Postnatal depression can be a difficult subject to broach. Clients may not wish to contemplate such 'gloom and doom' when they are looking forward to a happy event. The causes of postnatal depression are not yet fully understood but are almost certainly multifactorial.[7] An antenatal teacher cannot prevent it, but you should encourage a woman to discuss her feelings with her partner, other mothers and her midwife or health visitor. When suffering in this way it is a strengthening comfort to know one is not mad, and not alone. Constructive advice to help her plan to avoid tiredness is also useful. Since depressed people often do not seek the help they need, it is necessary for partners to be able to recognize the need for assistance.

Resuming sexual intercourse after the birth will depend on individual physical and emotional factors and clients can be helped to resume a happy and fulfilling relationship with their partners if they do not aim for some non-existent norm. Patience, consideration, maybe some practical advice and often humour are needed. Practical tips about positions and lubricating gel may be helpful for the early days or weeks when tender perinea and breasts are troublesome.

Contraception could be discussed. Mothers may feel the subject remote while they are still pregnant. If not encouraged to make preparations soon after the birth, they may be returning sooner than anticipated! They may not realize that ovulation and therefore fertility returns before menstruation.

(c) TAKING BABY HOME

Going home with a new baby means huge physical, emotional and social adjustments. '*Looking forward to getting back to normal*' is a phrase sometimes used by pregnant mothers or their partners. It may be a form of normality, but life will never be the same again! If mothers believe in the glamorous image of motherhood portrayed by the media,

Life After Birth

they are likely to find the reality a great shock. The realization of what parenthood means may take time to sink in even when it has been discussed antenatally. It can be helpful if you can encourage them to consider some practical aspects. Tiredness is a complaint of most new mothers. Ask your clients to think about possible sources of help available to them when they return home. Also, how they can make the most of the help that is available. If mother-in-law is coming to stay, she can be encouraged to do the washing and cooking rather than look after the baby. If friends offer help, the mother can have a list of jobs or shopping that needs doing ready to hand. Ask them to consider their priorities: a contented baby and a rested mother, or a tidy clean house and a pile of perfectly ironed clothes. Ask clients to think about visitors, whether they will expect to be entertained or will go and make themselves and the mother a cup of tea (and wash up afterwards). If the mother wishes to control visitors, she could write on the birth announcement cards times when visitors will be welcome, or even pin a note on the front door. Advise the mother how to save time and effort on cooking. If she has a freezer, she could stock it up before the birth. The family's diet will not seriously suffer if they eat a few take-away meals.

When mothers return home from hospital will depend, in part, on the health of herself and the baby, and in part on the policies of the hospital. If she is allowed to choose, ask her to consider if it is better for her to remain in hospital where she has no domestic responsibilities and where help is available for breast feeding. Or she may relax and rest better and feel more confident in her own home environment. It will be helpful for a mother to know she will continue to receive care from a midwife and then a health visitor after she returns home.

Think about what advice you can give mothers about dealing with their own and their partners' changing roles and feelings (see Chapter 4). Hearing about how others have felt,

Life After Birth

what problems they experienced and what solutions they found may not cover every eventuality, but it may encourage them to find their own ways of coping. It can also help them to realize the range of adjustments which may be needed. There may be big changes in lifestyle, change in working day (and night!) and adaptation of their social life. Contact with other mothers is important – it is possible to feel very lonely at home with a new baby. The antenatal classes themselves may be a source of social contacts after the birth. You could give the clients information about local groups such as mother-and-baby clubs or postnatal support groups or National Childbirth Trust groups.

If you have second-time mothers attending, you could discuss how the older child will adjust to the new baby. Jealousy can be a problem but may be avoided with forethought. Even simple measures such as the baby not being in the mother's arms when the toddler first sees her after the birth, or giving a present *from* the baby to the sibling may be useful.

You could revise what you have previously taught about material preparations for baby. A reminder about safety factors may be appropriate at this time (see Chapter 5). You may feel it appropriate to give clients information about how to obtain the birth certificate and how to register the baby with a general practitioner.

(d) ROLE OF THE HEALTH VISITOR

Whether or not you are able to invite a health visitor to the classes, it is useful to discuss how she can help clients. Most mothers have heard of health visitors but many have a distorted idea of their role. Clients sometimes see health visitors as interfering snoopers instead of the supportive friends they often become. The health visitor will monitor the progress of the baby and you could talk about the development checks she or the doctor will carry out. This is also a suitable time to

Life After Birth

introduce the subject of immunization. The uptake of immunization is not as great as health authorities wish and it is helpful if midwives can put forward a positive viewpoint. Also, it is useful to give mothers the opportunity to voice any worries they may have about possible adverse effects of vaccines. The whooping cough vaccine is the one which causes most concern to mothers and while between 1 and 5 per cent of children may have contra-indications to it, parents can sometimes receive conflicting advice.[8] You may be able to tell them the official policy of the health district in which you work and the criteria that are used to make decisions about whether or not to immunize.

(e) POSTNATAL EXAMINATION

The importance of the postnatal examination at six weeks after the birth could be discussed. Mothers can be encouraged not to consider this as the absolute finale of childbirth. All physical problems may not have been fully resolved, for example, a sutured perineum may continue to cause pain. Postnatal depression may still require treatment and possibly may not even have been diagnosed. If the postnatal examination is seen by the mother as the end of professional interest in her, she may fail to ask for any help she needs. You could encourage her to voice her concerns about painful sex, stress incontinence or feelings of not coping and to see them as valid. In this way maximum benefit can be obtained from a routine examination which is often undervalued.[9]

(f) ....

Can you think of anything else clients may need or want to know?

Life After Birth

4 How Will You Teach?

Discussion can bring out many points you wish to cover and possibly some you had not thought of. These latter points may be of vital importance to the client, however trivial they may appear to you. Many clients may have friends or relatives who have talked of emotions after birth, or a painful perineum, or postnatal depression, and if you 'ask' instead of 'tell', much valuable information will be shared.

Exercises are most easily learned by demonstration and practice.

A demonstration of how best to achieve a comfortable sitting position with a painful sutured perineum may help them to remember this advice post-delivery, if it is necessary.

You need to think about whether these subjects should be covered at one or more sessions or if more than one person will be involved. Hospital midwife, community midwife, obstetric physiotherapist and health visitor could all have an input. Think about how you will liaise to ensure that neither conflicting advice nor too much repetition occurs.

5 What Aids Will You Use?

A mother invited to come to the class or a video of mothers discussing their experiences can stimulate discussion on feelings and practical matters.

Advice for teaching postnatal exercises is available in a reprint of an article by an obstetric physiotherapist in the *Midwives Chronicle*.[10] A more comprehensive programme is described in a book giving a six-month programme of graded exercises.[11]

Life After Birth

6 Trigger Questions for Discussion

How do you expect to feel emotionally/physically immediately after the birth?
What have friends told you about how they felt in the first few days after the birth?
How do you see your life changing at home with a new baby?
What help do you expect to get from partner/mother/friends?
How will you feel about visitors when you are in hospital/when you return home?
What sort of routine would you expect yourself and your baby to be in at two weeks old?
What do you expect to have to do to get back to a shape and weight that satisfies you?
To multiparae:
   Can you remember how you felt just after the birth?
   How did you feel when you took your baby home?

7 How Will You Know When You Have Done It?

Feedback during the class will give you some idea whether or not you are getting your message across. Useful assessment and evaluation can be obtained by interviewing clients after the birth. This could be anything from a friendly chat to a formal questionnaire.

A reunion class can also be helpful to both the teacher and clients, providing an opportunity to discuss, and hopefully, resolve negative feelings about the experience. The Edinburgh Postnatal Depression Scale, while not an evaluation of your teaching, could be used at a postnatal reunion to discover those mothers who might benefit from further help.[12]

Life After Birth

Suggested Leaflets

From Association of Chartered Physiotherapists in Obstetrics and Gynaecology/Milupa:

Postnatal exercises and advice.

From Family Planning Association/Health Education Authority:

When you've had your baby.

From Health Education Authority:

Immunisation. Information for Parents.
MMR. Give your child something you never had.

From National Childbirth Trust:

Sex in pregnancy and after childbirth.

References

1 Sleep, J. and Grant, A. (1987), 'Salt in bathwater', *Research and the Midwife*, Conference Proceedings, pp. 65–75.
2 National Childbirth Trust (1988), *A Survey of Postnatal Infection*, NCT, London.
3 Romito, P. (1986), 'The humanising of childbirth: the response of medical institutions to women's demands for change', *Midwifery*, vol. 2, no. 2, September, pp. 135–40.
4 Gordon, H. and Logue, M. (1985), 'Perineal muscle function after childbirth', *The Lancet*, vol. 2, 20 July, pp. 123–5.
5 Jackson, W. (1988), 'New generation', *NCT*, vol. 7, no. 1, March, pp. 20–1.
6 Attwood, G. (1988), 'Motherlove – do midwives help or hinder?', Presentation to the Forum on Maternity and the Newborn at the Royal Society of Medicine, 24 February. In *MIDIRS*, no. 9, November 1988.

7 Cox, J. L. (1986), *Postnatal Depression. A Guide for Health Professionals*, Churchill Livingstone, Edinburgh, pp. 33–52.
8 Ross, E. M. (1986), 'Whooping cough vaccination – getting the balance right', *Maternal and Child Health*, vol. 11, no. 12, December, pp. 382–5.
9 Bowers, J. (1985), 'Is the six-weeks postnatal examination necessary?' *The Practitioner*, vol. 229, pp. 1113–5.
10 Polden, M. (1985), 'Teaching postnatal exercises', *Midwives Chronicle*, vol. 98, no. 1173, October, pp. 271–4.
11 Whiteford, B. and Polden, M. (1988), *Postnatal Exercises. A Six Month Fitness Programme for Mother and Baby*, 2nd edn, Century, London.
12 Cox, *Postnatal Depression. A Guide for Health Professionals*, pp. 20, 21, 85 and 86.

Further Reading

Ball, J. A. (1987), *Reactions to Motherhood*, Cambridge University Press, Cambridge.

Bull, M. and Lawrence, D. (1985), 'Mothers' Use of Knowledge During the first Postpartum Weeks', *Journal of Obstetric, Gynaecological and Neonatal Nurses*, vol. 14, no. 4, July/August, pp. 315–20.

Appendix 1 Resources

Books and journals are an obvious resource but you need to know where to find them. There are many professional libraries that may be available to you. You will need to discover what facilities there are in your own area. Your local hospital may have a School of Nursing or Medical College library. The local Health Education Department may have relevant books and journals. If libraries are too far away for you to visit, some may be able to supply photocopies of journal articles. Most libraries will have photocopying facilities available for you to use when you visit, but do take care to stay within the laws of copyright.

Professional Libraries

Health Education Authority Library (previously Health Education Council)
   Hamilton House
   Mabledon Place
   London WC1H 9TX
   You may join and borrow books
Health Visitors Association Library
   50 Southark Street
   London SE1
   Members may borrow books, non-members may read there
Kings Fund Library
   126 Albert Street

Appendix 1 Resources

London NW1
Reading in library only
Royal College of Midwives Library
15 Mansfield Street
London W1
Members may borrow books, non-members may read there
Royal College of Nursing Library
20 Cavendish Square
London W1
Members only
Your local Health Education/Promotion Unit: a resource centre for advice, books, leaflets, teaching packs, slides, videos and films; assistance with graphics

HOW TO USE YOUR HEALTH EDUCATION DEPARTMENT

Introduce yourself and make an appointment. Health education officers are busy people and may not be able to see you if you arrive unannounced. Let them know in advance what your needs are, whether it is to find out what is available or to seek help with a particular project. This may affect who you see – there may be a health education officer with responsibility for your field. Give them some idea of the amount of time you require. Overestimate required time rather than underestimate – ten minutes usually escalates to thirty. Allow adequate time when ordering materials. Return borrowed items promptly. Resources are free.

Useful Addresses and Resources

Association of Breastfeeding Mothers
131 Mayow Road
Sydenham
London SE26 4HZ
Leaflets and members newsletter, telephone and group support to clients

Appendix 1 Resources

Association of British Insurers (ABI)
  Aldermary House
  Queen Street
  London EC4N 1TT
  Leaflet and film on home safety

Association of Chartered Physiotherapists in Obstetrics and Gynaecology (APCOG)
  14 Bedford Row
  London W1
  Members of this Association often cover the physical preparation of mothers in antenatal classes but also run courses to assist midwives who have to undertake this; you should be able to make contact through your local hospital

Association for the Improvement of Maternity Services (AIMS)
  19 Broomfield Crescent
  Leeds 6
  A voluntary pressure group; gives support and advice to clients

Association for Postnatal Illness
  7 Gowan Avenue
  Fulham
  London SW6
  Advice and support to mothers suffering from postnatal depression

AIDS Education and Research Trust (AVERT)
  PO Box 91
  Horsham
  West Sussex RH13 7YR
  Leaflet: *AIDS and Childbirth*

Bear Necessities Directory
  Bridget Spowart
  Pandora Publishing
  42 Eaton Crescent
  Swansea SA1 4QL

Appendix 1   Resources

A book listing a wide variety of suppliers (often mail order) of baby equipment; also lists many support groups of interest to pregnant and new mothers

BBC Enterprises
 Villiers House
 The Broadway
 London W5
 Health and social studies videos; guidance notes for childbirth educators, for use with the *Having a Baby* series

British Standards Institution
 Public Relations Department
 2 Park Street
 London WIA 2
 Information on safety of manufactured goods; leaflet on British Standards in baby and child equipment

Child Accident Prevention Trust
 28 Portland Place
 London WIN 4DE
 Leaflets and videos

Childbirth Graphics Ltd.
 1210 Culver Road
 Rochester
 New York, USA, 14609–5454
 Wide variety of visual aids

Commission for Racial Equality
 Elliot House
 10–12 Allington Street
 London SW1E 5EH
 Antenatal language kit, to teach English for pregnancy

Cow and Gate
 Trowbridge
 Wiltshire, BA14 8HZ
 Films, leaflets and posters; teaching aids on pregnancy, birth and feeding – *A New Life*, flip chart or slide set

Appendix 1   Resources

CRY-SIS
B. M. CRY-SIS
London WCIN 3XX
Support group for parents of babies who cry excessively

Department of Health and Social Security
  Leaflets Unit
  PO Box 21
  Stanmore
  Middlesex
  Leaflets on benefits for mothers and babies
  Drugs in Breast Milk Information service (DIBMIS)
  Access through your local Hospital Drug Information Unit

Equipment for the Disabled
  Mary Marlborough Lodge
  Nuffield Orthopaedic Centre
  Headington
  Oxford OX3 7LD
  Books, including *Equipment for the Disabled Mother*

Family Planning Association
  27–35 Mortimer Street
  London WIA 4QW
  Leaflets, posters and advice to clients

Farley Health Products Ltd
  Torr Lane
  Plymouth
  Devon
  Leaflets and posters

Plymouth Medical Films
  33 New Street
  The Barbican
  Plymouth PLI 2NA
  Videos, films and slides for hire or sale

Appendix 1   Resources

Foresight, The Association of Preconceptual Care
  Woodhurst
  Hydestile
  Godalming
  Surrey
  Advice to clients; newsletter to members; leaflets and books
Graves Medical Audiovisual Library
  Holly House
  220 New London Road
  Chelmsford
  Essex CM2 9BJ
  Videos and tape/slide sets
Health Education Authority (previously Health Education Council),
  Hamilton House
  Mabledon Place
  London WC1H 9TX
  Leaflets and posters, usually available through your local
Health Education Unit
  La Leche League
  PO Box BM2434
  London WC1 6
  Leaflets, advice to clients
Meet-a-mum Association (MAMA)
  3 Woodside Avenue
  South Norwood
  London SE25
Maternity Alliance
  59–61 Camden High Street
  London NW1 7JL
  Leaflets, advice to clients
Midwives Information and Resource Service (MIDIRS),
  Institute of Child Health
  Royal Hospital for Sick Children
  St Michael's Hill
  Bristol BS2 8BJ

Appendix 1 Resources

Subscribing members receive three information packs each year; there is also an enquiry service; run by midwives for midwives to enable them to improve and update their practice

Milupa Ltd
  Milupa House
  Uxbridge Road
  Hillingdon
  Uxbridge
  Middlesex UB10 0NE
  Films, videos, leaflets, mini pelvis with fetal doll.

Mothercare
  Sylvia Meredith
  Health Education Advisory Service
  3 Elgin Road
  Sutton
  Surrey
  Leaflets and posters

National Childbirth Trust
  Alexandra House
  Oldhan Terrace
  London W3 6NH
  Advice to clients through antenatal classes, postnatal support groups and breastfeeding counsellors, leaflets, posters, and books; sales and fitting of nursing bras, sales of clothes and baby equipment

National Council for Civil Liberties
  Rights for Women Unit
  21 Tabard Street
  London SE1 4LA
  Voluntary pressure group; leaflets and books; advice to clients

Open University
  Learning Materials Service Office
  PO Box 188
  Milton Keynes MK7 6DH

Appendix 1 Resources

Teaching materials, including *Understanding Pregnancy and Birth, a Teaching Pack* (1987)

Royal National Institute for the Blind
  Bakewell Road
  Orton Southgate
  Peterborough
  Cambridgeshire PE2 0XU
  Catalogue of resources; braille books, audio tapes, useful addresses

Royal National Institute for the Deaf
  105 Gower Street
  London WC1
  Leaflets on communicating with the deaf (including basic sign language) and special baby equipment

Royal Society for the Prevention of Accidents (ROSPA)
  Head Office, Cannon House
  Priory Queensway
  Birmingham
  Leaflets and advice

Rycote Centre for the Deaf
  Parker Street
  Derby DE1 3HF
  Booklet of sign language for use in relaxation and labour

Twins and Multiple Births Association (TAMBA)
  Jenny Smith, Secretary
  41 Fortuna Way
  Aylesby Park
  Grimsby
  South Humberside DN37 9SJ
  Leaflets and books; group support for clients

Teaching Aids at Low Cost
  PO Box 49
  St Albans
  Herts AL1 4AX

Appendix 1 Resources

Books and slide sets
Vegan Society
  33–35 George Street
  Oxford OX1 2AY
  Leaflets and books
Vegetarian Society
  Parkdale
  Dunhan
  Altringham
  Cheshire WA14 4QG
  Leaflets and books
Wyeth Laboratories
  Taplow
  Maidenhead
  Berkshire
  Leaflets and posters, films

This list is not exhaustive; many of the organizations listed will provide further information and teaching aids.

The book *Antenatal Education, Guidelines for Teachers* by Williams and Booth reviews a large selection of the films, videos and slides.

Beware of unwanted advertising with some commercial materials.

Prices of hiring or buying equipment have not been included as these would inevitably rise and become out of date.

Appendix 2 What Next?

This book does not pretend to tell you all you need to know. The analogy of the book as a lifeline to those midwives thrown in at the deep end is perhaps misleading. A lifeline implies that all you have to do is to grab the lifeline, reach the end and all will be finished. Not so with teaching: to begin teaching is to begin a journey that will last as long as you teach. It will sometimes be uphill, but will have its rewards.

Further study will help you to improve your skills and maintain your enthusiasm. The journal articles and books listed at the end of each chapter are not merely there to prove this book has been researched, they are there to be read. Keep your eye on professional journals for recent research.

Do not dismiss books as irrelevant because the title suggests they have little to do with your particular field. *How Children Fail* contains some thought-provoking material on the learning process and what hinders it. You may feel that a study of psychotherapy is not necessary for an antenatal teacher, but Carl Rogers has some pertinent things to say about personal relationships and their effect on learning. Knowledge of the psychology of learning and of the psychological factors that affect childbirth will enhance your practice. Many of the articles and books listed contain bibliographies that will suggest further reading.

Appendix 2   What Next?

Courses of Study

Listed below are some courses which can help you to increase your proficiency as an antenatal teacher. Courses which draw students from different fields can provide valuable sharing of ideas and experience. This allows a student to stand back from her own teaching situation and take in a wider view of teaching and learning.

I   CITY AND GUILDS OF LONDON COURSE 7307, FURTHER AND ADULT EDUCATION TEACHERS' CERTIFICATE

(a) Qualification and selection of students
Selection of students is at the discretion of the college and its controlling authority. Students may come from many disciplines, including education, medicine, commerce, industry and public service. Applicants would normally be accepted if they already held a qualification relevant to their job and were, or were about to become, involved in training or teaching as part of that job.

(b) Cost
This varies considerably from college to college. It will consist in part of college fees and in part of a certification fee payable to the City and Guilds of London Institute. Certification fees for 1989 – £28.20p. College fees: £80 upwards.

(c) Venue
Courses are offered at about 200 centres throughout England and Wales. A list of colleges is available from:
City and Guilds of London Institute
46 Britannia Street
London WC1X 9RG

Appendix 2 What Next?

(d) Length and structure of course

The course is part-time, based on the academic year for one or two years. It is divided into two stages. The purposes of stage one are introductory and exploratory and it lasts for forty hours. Stage two extends and develops the work and lasts for 130 hours. This adds up to a minimum of 170 hours of study and practice. There will be a minimum of thirty hours' teaching practice, of which a minimum of twelve hours will be supervised.

(e) Aims

The major aims of the course are:

To introduce teachers to the principles of learning.

To enable teachers to make a conscious choice of teaching methods based on an understanding of learning principles.

To enable teachers to evaluate and use effectively the resources available to themselves and students.

To enable teachers to design appropriate programmes, courses, schemes of work with the active participation of the learning group.

To enable teachers to understand principles and methods of assessment, and in particular to relate these effectively to the aims and objectives of the course they are teaching.

To develop the abilities of teachers to communicate in order to enhance their own effectiveness as educators and to enable them to assist students to develop their own communication abilities.

To enable teachers to make effective appraisals of their own professional roles, responsibilities and teaching styles.

(f) Course content

The subjects covered include the principles of learning and teaching, learning resources, course organization and curriculum development, assessment, communication and the role of the teacher. There is a core element laid down by the

Appendix 2 What Next?

institute and an element designed by each college. Assignments will include written work on the theory and practice of teaching. Students will be required to design and make audio-visual or visual aids.

The teaching study is the major assignment in which the student will:

Identify a learning group.
Analyse and describe the group.
Observe and evaluate the performance of an experienced teacher conducting this or a comparable group.
Plan, present and evaluate a lesson with the group.
Design, use and evaluate a teaching programme with the group.
Identify and comment on principles of learning demonstrated during the teaching of this programme.
Design, use and evaluate teaching aids.
Identify and comment on teaching methods used.
Identify and analyse problems of communication encountered.
Write or present an in-depth study of an educational issue associated with the chosen teaching programme.

The local college element will provide the tutor with the opportunity to relate to the individual student's needs, skills and particular areas of professional concern.

(g) Assessment
There is continuous assessment with the emphasis on the student's performance as a teacher. The process of marking students' written work and the assessment of teaching practice is seen less as a grading exercise and more as an opportunity for constructive critical comment and discussion.

A personal profile will be negotiated between tutor and student and will include essential details of the course and student, teaching experience gained during the course and

Appendix 2 What Next?

characteristics of the student's performance. Personal details may be given where these have a bearing on future development and show evidence of the student's capacity for self-evaluation.

(h) Certificate
The course is validated by the City and Guilds of London Institute, which issues a certificate of performance to successful candidates. Grade is 'pass' only.

2 HEALTH EDUCATION CERTIFICATE

(a) Qualification and selection of students
Each college will consider individual applications. Students are required to have a basic professional qualification and experience in one of the health, social work, environmental health, industrial health or voluntary services.

Cost
Each college sets its own fees, so this will vary. Average 1989 fee: £189.

(c) Venue
Courses are offered at about forty-one colleges throughout England, Wales and Northern Ireland. List of colleges available from:
Health Education Authority
Hamilton House
Mabledon Place
London WC1H 9TX

(d) Length and structure of course
The organization of the course will vary in different colleges. The usual structure is one day each week for one academic year. A number of colleges include short blocks of teaching, sometimes on a residential basis. Five colleges offer an open learning mode.

Appendix 2 What Next?

(e) Aims

To enable students to extend and develop their professional communication skills and techniques and be aware of attitudes, behaviour and priorities in relation to their particular health education practice. To provide opportunities for the student to use and evaluate the various strategies in real and simulated practice.

(f) Course content

The content will include those aspects of social and behavioural sciences, social medicine, political and educational theory which are seen to be relevant to the practice of health education. Subjects covered will include models of health education, sociological perspectives of health/illness, research, learning theories and processes, working with groups, epidemiology, politics of health, designing health education programmes, evaluation of teaching materials, communication skills and assertiveness skills.

Written work may include an essay and a literature review. The major assignment is an in-depth study which may be a research project or the development of a teaching aid. Practical work will include making visual aids and supervised teaching practice. This will take place partly in college within the group and partly in the student's own professional teaching situation.

(g) Assessment

There will be continuous assessment of the student's performance in written and practical work. The institutions appoint an approved external assessor, drawn from the Register of External Assessors held by the Certificate Course Board.

(h) Certificate

The course is validated by the Health Education Authority which issues a certificate to successful candidates.

Appendix 2 What Next?

3 NATIONAL CHILDBIRTH TRUST ANTENATAL TEACHER TRAINING

(a) Qualification and selection of students
Students are lay but some are professional; all have borne children. They are expected to be a member of and have a basic knowledge and acceptance of the attitudes and aims of NCT. Prospective students will be interviewed by a local tutor and on her recommendation will be accepted for training.

(b) Cost
Fees are payable for study days and from May 1989 a small charge will be made for tutorials and workshops. Students are expected to pay any expenses incurred. Financial support may be available from local NCT branches.

(c) Training
This is possible anywhere in the country that tutors are available. Training is usually in the tutor's home. Application can be made through a local NCT branch or by writing to:
National Childbirth Trust Headquarters
Alexandra House
Oldham Terrace
London W3 6NH

(d) Length and structure of course
A student will serve a probationary period of at least six months and then become a registered student. The training is flexible to allow a student to work at her own pace and according to her other work or family commitments. Most students will take between 1½ and 2½ years to qualify.

(e) Aims
The NCT sees its teachers as group leaders rather than

Appendix 2 What Next?

conventional teachers. The aim is to prepare them for their role in supporting parents through pregnancy, labour, birth and early parenthood.

(f) Course content

Subjects will include normal and abnormal pregnancy, labour, birth and the puerperium. This will cover psychological aspects and involvement of the mother's partner, current issues of choice in childbirth and cultural differences. Also included are teaching methods, communication skills, group dynamics, audio-visual aids, counselling skills, relationships with professionals and self-development. The practicalities of starting a class are taught, including bookings, records, finance, legal liability and the Data Protection Act.

During the probationary period the student will sit in on a course of antenatal classes given by an experienced teacher who will be nominated by the tutor. The tutor will also ask the student to read certain books and will set some written work. At least six months' involvement with branch activities is required. After the student becomes registered she will observe a second, different course of antenatal classes and continue written work set by the tutor. She will attend two teaching workshops and any study days that are recommended by her tutor.

(g) Assessment

There is continuous assessment by the tutor of the student's performance. Written work to be assessed will be an essay on a subject agreed with the tutor and a teaching plan. These are submitted to a teacher's panel. If the work is accepted the student becomes an accredited teacher. She is then asked to write an assessment of her whole training. Each teacher will have her teaching reviewed at regular intervals.

(h) Certificate

The NCT issues a certificate upon accreditation of the teacher.

Appendix 2   What Next?

Others courses that are available include The Royal College of Midwives: Preparation for Parenthood Educators (Apply to: The Royal College of Midwives, 15 Mansfield Street, London WIM OBE) and ENB 997, Teaching in Clinical Practice (Apply to your school of nursing).

Your local Health Education Department may also run short courses on specific subjects, such as communication or use of visual aids.

An antenatal teacher may find herself working in isolation. Contact with other antenatal teachers can provide support and stimulation. This may happen on a regular basis within your district: if it does not, you may be able to suggest that teachers get together to share their knowledge, feelings and problems. Parent Educators Group Support (PEGS) meets regularly at RCM headquarters. PEGS can advise on setting up a group in your area.

Index

activity in learning, 11, 15, 18–20
adoptive parents, 29
affective domain, 4, 16
aims and objectives for teaching, 1–6, 10, 35
    partners, 55–6; pregnancy, 71–2; relaxation and breathing for labour, 93–4; labour and birth, 112–13; baby care and feeding, 140–1; life after birth, 169–70
alcohol:
    and baby in parental bed, 158
    in pregnancy, 59, 75
    during breastfeeding, 150
analysis of classroom activity, 10–11
antenatal care, 81–3
    partner's role in, 59–60
assessment of learning, 1, 6–10
    self, 10
attendance at classes, 27–8
attitudes, 5, 11, 15, 35, 65, 118

baby:
    capabilities of newborn, 156–7
    care, 5, 27
    by mother, 155–8; by midwife, 158–9; by paediatrician, 159–60
    crying, 157–8
    equipment, *see* layette
    resuscitation, 64
benefits, 85
birth plan, 129
body language, 11, 37–8
bonding, 156–7, 171
bottle-feeding:
    choice of formula, 152–3, 154
    sterilization of equipment, 153
    theory and practice, 152–3
breastfeeding:
    appearance of baby's stools, 149
    brassières for, 150–1
    effect on mother's figure, 144–5, 149–50
    factors for success, 148
    fixing baby, 148
    'let down' reflex, 147–8
    mother's diet during, 149
    partner's role in, 142, 145
    patterns of, 151–2
    preparation for, 146–7
    and return to work, 145, 154–5

Index

sources of advice, 154
theory and practice, 146–52
breast milk:
  immunological significance, 143, 152
breathing:
  abdominal, 100
  for labour, 63, 101–2, 121–2
    first stage, 102–3;
    second stage, 104–5, 117
buzz group, 31

carpal tunnel syndrome, 57, 79
client need, 13, 22, 26–7, 28–9
cognitive domain, 4, 16
conditioning, 14–5
cramp, 76
criticism, 11, 20, 22, 38, 142

demonstration, 6, 32
diet:
  in pregnancy, 4, 73–4
  in labour, 126–7
  during breastfeeding, 149
disability, 29
discussion, 6, 10, 20, 30–1
  concluding, 41
  getting started, 36–7
  keeping going, 37–8
  problem members in, 39–40
  trigger questions for:
    baby care and feeding, 163–4; labour and birth, 135; life after birth, 180; partners, 68–9; pregnancy, 87; relaxation and breathing for labour, 109; reunion class, 9–10
drugs:
  in pregnancy, 75
  in labour, 122–5
  during breastfeeding, 150

emotions:
  after birth, 64
  in labour, 63
  in pregnancy, 58
entonox, 103, 125
environmental hazards:
  in pregnancy, 82
  during breastfeeding, 144
epidural anaesthesia, 116, 124–5, 131
episiotomy, 128
evaluation of teaching, 1, 10
exercise:
  in pregnancy, 76–7
exercises:
  abdominal, 77, 173
  pelvic floor, 77–8, 173, 179
fatherhood:
  attitudes to, 65
  feedback, 6, 11–2
fetal:
  development, 72–3
  monitoring, 127
films, *see* video

group work:
  concluding, 41
  facilitating discussion, 36–7
  leadership, 35, 37
  planning, 34–5
  problem members, 39–41
  seating, 35
  size, 34
  venue, 34–5

Index

hazards, *see also* environmental
  in the home, 84–5
health education:
  models, 2
  department, 184
health educators, role of, 125, 126
health visitor, 49, 133, 177–8
hyperventilation, 101, 103

immunization, 178
infant feeding, *see also* breast and bottle feeding:
  advantages and disadvantages of methods, 142–6
  choice of method, 141–2
  positions for, 162

knitted uterus, 44–5

labour:
  abnormal, 129–31
  breathing for, 63, 100–5, 121
  companion, 61–4
  coping strategies for, 5, 118–22
  diet in, 126–7
  massage in, 63, 122
  medical intervention in, 129–31
  mobility in, 119–20, 121
  pain in, 118
  pain relief for, 122–5
  partner's role in, 61–4, 128, 130
  physiology of, 115–18
  policies and procedures, 63, 125–9
  positions in, 77, 117, 119–21, 128
  second stage, 104–5, 117–18
  signs of, 113–15
  teaching in, 122
  third stage, 118
language:
  use of 8, 16, 17, 75, 115
  problems, 29
layette, 83–4
leadership, 35–6, 37
leaflets, 49, 69, 88–9, 136, 164–5, 181
learning:
  activity in, 11, 15–16
  definition of, 13
  and memory, 18
  motivation for, 13
  responsibility for, 23
  theories of, 14–16
Leboyer birth, 128
lecture, 30
lesson plans, 50–1
libraries, 183–4
ligaments:
  in pregnancy, 57, 78–9
  after birth, 64, 78

memory, 18
metaphors, 16–17
morning sickness, 57, 76

nicotine:
  effect on fetus, 74
  in breast milk, 150
nipple:
  care, 146–7
  stimulation, 61, 130
nutrition, *see* diet

Index

objectives, *see* aims and objectives
one-to-one teaching, 29, 34
overhead projector, 42–3, 47

pain:
  in labour, 118
  relief, 5, 122–5
pantograph, 43–4
partners:
  after birth, 64–5
  attitudes to infant feeding, 142, 145, 147
  in classes, 66
  in labour and birth, 61–4, 128, 130
  needs, 56–7
  in pregnancy, 57–61
  relaxation, 61
pelvic floor, *see* exercises
pelvic floor model, 45–7
perception, 13–14, 17, 21–2, 28
perineal care, 170–1, 178
pethidine, 103, 122
physiotherapist, obstetric, 49, 76, 79, 133, 173
placenta, 73, 174
planning checklist, 51–2
posters, 35, 49
postnatal:
  depression, 64–5, 174–5
  examination, 64, 178
posture, 78
  of tension, 96
practical teaching, 32
pregnancy:
  alcohol in, 59, 75
  diet in, 4, 73–4, 76
  emotions, 58, 79–80
  exercise in, 76–7
  ligaments in, 57, 78–9
  minor disorders of, 57, 76, 79
  partner's feelings in, 57–8
  rights and benefits, 85
  sex in, 60–1, 79–80
  smoking in, 59, 74
  travel in, 82
  wearing of car seat belts, 79
problem solving, 15–6, 31–2
prostaglandins, 61
psychomotor domain, 4
puerperium:
  physical care in, 170–4
  emotions, 174–5

questionnaires, 6–9
questions, 6, 19–20, 38, 81, 83, *see also* discussion, trigger

relationships:
  client/carer, 126
  learner/learner, 37
  mother/baby, 156–7, 171
  mother/partner, 60, 64, 67, 80, 176
  teacher/learner, 16, 21–3
relaxation:
  breathing in, 100
  choice of method, 94–6
  in labour, 121
  mental, 99–100
  Mitchell method, 96–9
  partners, 61
  positions for, 106
  reciprocal, 96
  touch in, 67, 95
relevance in learning, 17, 28, 38
reunion of antenatal class, 9–10

Index

rewards and punishments, 20
role play, 33, 67, 132

safety:
   in the car, 85
   in the home, 83–5
sex:
   after birth, 175
   during breastfeeding, 147–8
   in pregnancy, 60–1, 79–80
siblings, 177
smoking:
   in pregnancy, 59, 74
   during breastfeeding, 150
social contact at classes, 27
squatting, 77, 116
stimulus/response, 00

teaching aids, 41–9, 86, 108, 133–5, 163, 179
   knitted uterus, 44–5
teaching methods, 29–34
teaching notes, 51

teenage parents, 29
toxoplasmosis, 82
transcutaneous electrical nerve stimulation, 123–4
trial and error learning, 15–16, 31–2
trigger questions, *see* questions

Ultrasound scanning, 82

Valsalva manoeuvre, 104
venue for classes, 34–5
video and films, 48, 68
visits, 33, 67
visual aids, *see* teaching aids

weight:
   after birth, 149–50
   in pregnancy, 73
words, *see* language

Yoga, 77, 94, 104